Susannah James

Recipes For The Eight Week
Blood Sugar Diet

First Published 2017

Published by Lionheart Publishing

Copyright © 2017 Lionheart Publishing

All rights reserved. No part of this book shall be reproduced, stored in a retrieval system, or transmitted by any means, electronic, mechanical, recording, photocopying or otherwise, without the prior written permission of the publisher.

Notice of Liability

A great deal of effort has gone into ensuring that the content of this book is both accurate and up to date. However, Lionheart Publishing and the author will not be held liable for any loss or damage from the use of the information herein.

Trademarks

All trademarks are acknowledged as belonging to their respective companies.

Contents

Chapter One - Breakfast Recipes

French Omelette 12

Mushroom Quiche 13

Baked Eggs With Spinach 14

Power Porridge 15

Cinnamon Granola Bars 16

Egg and Leek Bake 17

Egg Ratatouille 18

Bircher Muesli 19

Scrambled Eggs 20

Kedgeree 21

Full English Breakfast 22

Almond Granola 23

Low-fat English Breakfast 24

Mushroom & Garlic Omelette 25

Apple and Linseed Porridge 26

Chapter Two - Lunch Recipes

Carrot Kugel ....

. 28

Chicken Burritos 29

Thai Cauliflower Rice 30

Duck Stir Fry 31

Salmon & Avocado Burger 32

Mushroom Penne 33

Poached Plaice 34

Spicy Avocado Wraps 35

Ginger Garlic Salmon 36

Lentil Curry 37

Oriental Steamed Fish 39

Thai Chilli Satay 40

Five-Spice Pork 41

Pakistani Chickpeas 42

Salmon Fish Cakes 43

Quinoa Pilaf 44

Chapter Three - Dinner Recipes

Jollof Chicken Rice 46

Prawn Biryani 48

Chicken & Chorizo Jambalaya 50

Sausage Stew 51

Venison Stir-Fry 52
Tandoori Chicken 53
Creamy Courgette Lasagne.. 54
Spicy Chicken & Broccoli Stir Fry 55
Pepper Ciambotta 56
Barbecue Pork Steaks 57
Chilli Casserole 58
Almond Nachos 59
Vegetable Paella 61
Chinese Braised Beef 63
Chicken And Leek Pie 65
Cauliflower Pizza 67
Beef Goulash 68
Nut Roast 70
Aubergine & Courgette Bake 72
Mushroom Risotto 73
Fish Stew 74
Chicken Fajitas 76

Chapter Four - Salad Recipes

Greek Salad 78
Couscous Salad 79

Quinoa Salad 80
Thai Chicken Salad 81
Lemon and Feta Salad.. 82
Squid and Pepper Salad 83
Vietnamese Beef Salad 84
Fire Salad 85
Indian Summer Salad 86
Avocado and Sunflower Salad 87
Sausage Salad 88

Chapter Five - Soup Recipes

Lentil & Bacon Soup 90
Chickpea Soup 91
Chilli Bean Soup 92
Bulgar Mushroom Soup 93
Minestrone Soup.. 95
Chicken Soup 96
Oriental Pumpkin Soup 97
Peanut Soup 98
Cauliflower Cheese Soup 99
Oriental Prawn Soup 100

Chapter Six - Snack Recipes

Cheesy Crisps 102

Pork & Pear Sausage Rolls 103

Quinoa Muffins 104

Feta Fritters 105

Lemon Houmous 106

Squash Chunks 107

Chicken Satay Pieces... 108

Salmon Mayonnaise Wraps 109

Chapter Seven - Dessert Recipes

Coconut Macaroons 112

Chocolate & Peanut Squares 113

Blueberry Ice Cream 114

Chocolate Fudge 115

Pumpkin Pie 116

Saffron Pannacotta 117

Berry Crumble.. 118

Lemon Squares 119

Introduction

An excess of sugar in the diet is, without doubt, the most serious health issue of our times. It is the main cause of the obesity epidemic currently sweeping the Western nations - the USA, UK, Australia and new Zealand in particular. In all of these countries, two-thirds of the adult population is now considered to be obese. Alarmingly, increasing numbers of children are going the same way.

Anyone who is overweight will have a high level of sugar in their blood. This has a drastic effect on their health. For starters, it vastly increases the risk of heart attacks and stroke. It is also very likely to lead to type 2 diabetes. If that's not bad enough, being overweight places a huge strain on every part of the body in general and ages people well before their time.

Excess blood sugar can damage both blood vessels and nerves in the body. This can result in poor blood flow to the hands, feet, arms, legs and vital organs. Quite apart from heart disease and stroke, the knock-on effects of this include increased risk of infections, blindness, foot or leg amputation and kidney disease. In addition, it can cause loss of feeling, and/or pain, in the feet and legs. In fact, serious damage to the feet can be caused by mild injuries with the person not even being aware of it. Finally, damage to blood vessels and nerves can lead to sexual problems that are difficult to treat effectively.

So, where does all this sugar come from? The answer is simple - the processed food industry. Virtually everything that comes out of a tin, packet or box is loaded with sugar. The solution is also simple. Cut refined sugar out of your diet! This means avoiding all processed food, and foods that are naturally high in sugar, such as tropical fruits - pineapples, mangoes, bananas and the like.

The recipes in this book are formulated to help you do just this. They rely on natural ingredients, avoid processed foods and will quickly bring your blood sugar under control. Not only will you look better, you will feel much, much better.

Breakfast Recipes

French Omelette 12
Mushroom Quiche 13
Baked Eggs With Spinach 14
Power Porridge 15
Cinnamon Granola Bars 16
Egg and Leek Bake 17
Egg Ratatouille 18
Bircher Muesli 19
Scrambled Eggs 20
Kedgeree 21
Full English Breakfast 22
Almond Granola 23
Low-fat English Breakfast 24
Mushroom & Garlic Omelette 25
Apple and Linseed Porridge 26

French Omelette

Chock-full of healthy ingredients, this omelette will give you the perfect start to the day.

<u>Serves 1</u>   <u>Prep time 5m</u>   <u>Cook time 10m</u>

1 mushroom
1 onion
1 clove garlic, minced
2 eggs
1 tsp basil
1 tbsp olive oil
1oz mozzarella cheese
1 tomato, chopped

Put the eggs and the basil in a bowl and whisk to a frothy consistency. Put to one side.

Then put the mushrooms, onion and garlic in a frying pan and fry them in the olive oil until cooked.

Add the egg and basil mixture to the frying pan over a medium heat and cook the omelette until it has set.

Sprinkle the mozzarella cheese over it, add the chopped tomato and serve.

Mushroom Quiche

The secret of this quiche is that it doesn't contain any pastry, i.e. carbohydrates.

Serves 4   **Prep time 15m**   **Cook time 30m**

300g mushrooms, coarsely chopped
1 onion, finely chopped
50g butter
2 tbsp dried breadcrumbs
2 tbsp parmesan cheese, grated
1/4 tsp black pepper, ground
100g cheddar cheese, grated
200g cream cheese
4 eggs
1 dash Tabasco Sauce
150g cooked ham or bacon, diced

In a medium pan, sauté the mushrooms and onion in the butter until just tender - about 5 minutes. Then stir in the breadcrumbs, parmesan cheese and pepper.

Butter the bottom and sides of a pie dish. Press the mushroom mix into the dish evenly on bottom and sides. Sprinkle the grated cheddar over the mixture.

In a blender (or by hand), beat the cream cheese, eggs and Tabasco sauce together until well mixed. Stir in the diced ham. Then pour the mixture over the mushrooms and cheese in the baking dish. Bake for 30 minutes.

Baked Eggs With Spinach

A hearty one-pot meal with a delicious combination of flavours. For a meatier dish, add chunks of cooked chicken, ham or bacon when you add the eggs.

<u>Serves 2</u>   <u>Prep time 10m</u>   <u>Cook time 40m</u>

200g new potatoes, thickly sliced
1 small onion, finely chopped
1 garlic clove, finely chopped
1/2 pepper, de-seeded and cut into small pieces
200g cannellini beans
2 medium tomatoes, chopped
150ml passata
1-2 tbsp Worcestershire sauce
50g spinach
2 eggs
1 handful of oregano

Boil the potatoes in a pan until they are tender and then drain them. Next, fry the onion, garlic and pepper in a frying pan for 5 minutes until they are soft.

Add them all to a large pan together with the beans, tomatoes, passata and Worcestershire sauce. Season and simmer for 10-12 minutes.

Stir in the spinach. Then make four small holes in the mixture and crack an egg into each one. Cover and cook for 5 minutes. Serve garnished with the oregano.

Power Porridge

Start your day with slow-release carbohydrates and plenty of fibre with this simple porridge.

<u>Serves 1</u>   <u>Prep time 5m</u>   <u>Cook time 5m</u>

75g quinoa
250ml water
250ml milk
2 apples, chopped finely or grated
1/2 tsp cinnamon
1 tsp vanilla extract
1 tbsp sunflower seeds
1 tbsp almonds, ground

Rinse the quinoa under cold running water and then mix it with the water in a pan. Bring to the boil and then reduce the heat. Cover and cook for 10 minutes until the quinoa is soft.

Add the milk, chopped apple, sunflower seeds, ground almonds, cinnamon and vanilla. Cook the porridge for 5 minutes until creamy. If necessary, add more milk for a creamier texture.

Ladle into a bowl and serve.

Cinnamon Granola Bars

These granola bars are great for lunch boxes, breakfast on the run or just with a cup of coffee.

<u>Makes 10</u>   <u>Prep time 15m</u>   <u>Cook time 30m</u>

100g butter
200g porridge oats
100g sunflower seeds
50g sesame seeds
50g walnuts, chopped
1 tsp honey
1 tsp cinnamon
100g mixed berries

Heat the oven to 160°C. Butter and line the base of a medium size baking tin. Mix the oats, seeds and walnuts in a roasting tin and then put them in the oven for 5-10 minutes to toast.

Next, melt the butter and honey in a pan. Add the oat mix, cinnamon and mixed berries, then mix until the oats are well coated.

Tip into the baking tin, compact the mixture lightly and then bake it for 30 minutes.

Allow to cool in the tin before cutting into 10 bars.

Egg and Leek Bake

This hearty country dish from the Provence region of France is an easy mix of seasonal vegetables, garlic and olive oil.

Serves 2   **Prep time 5m**   **Cook time 20m**

2 eggs
1 tsp olive oil
1/2 leek, thinly sliced
100g mushrooms, sliced
1 tbsp yogurt
Pinch of black pepper

Set the oven to 170°C. Put the oil in a frying pan and add the leeks and mushrooms. Stirring regularly, cook for 5 minutes.

Then mix in the yogurt and black pepper. When done, place the mixture in an oven-proof dish and bake for 15 minutes.

Remove from the oven and serve.

Egg Ratatouille

A simple and tasty breakfast that will fuel the whole family during the day to come.

<u>Serves 2</u>   <u>Prep time 10m</u>   <u>Cook time 50m</u>

2 eggs
1 pepper, de-seeded and thinly sliced
1 courgette, diced
1 tomato
1 onion, chopped
1 garlic clove, finely chopped
1 tbsp thyme
1 tbsp olive oil

Heat the oil in a large frying pan. Put the onion, pepper, garlic, courgette and thyme in the pan and fry for 3 minutes, stirring frequently.

Next, add the tomato and 200ml of water to the pan. Bring it to the boil, cover, and then simmer for 40 minutes.

Remove the ratatouille from the heat and make two spaces in it. Crack one egg into each space. Put it back on to a medium heat and let it cook for 5 minutes.

Then serve.

Bircher Muesli

Bircher Muesli was first made over a century ago by the Swiss doctor Maximilian Bircher-Benner in his Zurich clinic. It is traditionally left overnight to soften the oats.

Serves 1   Prep time 5m   Cook time 60m

25g rolled oats
1 tsp honey
100ml semi-skimmed milk
1 apple, unpeeled and grated
1 tbsp low-fat yogurt
10g walnuts, chopped
5 raspberries

Add the honey to the oats and then place into a pan with the milk. Leave to soak until all the milk has been absorbed (this should take about one hour), or overnight in the fridge.

Then mix the grated apple into the oats, and finish by putting the yogurt, raspberries and walnuts on top.

Scrambled Eggs

The key to making scrambled eggs is whisking the eggs thoroughly before cooking them. This incorporates air, which makes them lighter and fluffier.

<u>Serves 1</u>   <u>Prep time 5m</u>   <u>Cook time 5m</u>

3 eggs
1 mushroom
1 tomato
2 slices of ham
50ml milk
2 tsp butter

Place the eggs and milk in a bowl and whisk to a smooth consistency. Chop the tomato, mushroom and ham as finely as you can and stir them into the egg mixture.

Melt the butter in a frying pan and then add the egg mixture. With the pan on a medium heat, slowly cook it while stirring continuously.

Be careful not to overcook. The heat in the pan will continue to cook and firm up the eggs after they have been removed from heat.

When the scrambled egg is firm, it is ready to eat.

Kedgeree

This version of the breakfast classic is made with fresh salmon instead of smoked haddock, which is high in salt; and cauliflower instead of rice, which is high in carbohydrates.

<u>Serves 2</u>   <u>Prep time 10m</u>   <u>Cook time 30m</u>

1/2 cauliflower, grated
2 eggs
2 tsp olive oil
1 onion, finely chopped
150ml semi-skimmed milk
150g salmon
1 lemon, juice of
1 tbsp low-fat yogurt
2 tbsp cumin, finely chopped

Hard boil the eggs for twelve minutes or so, shell and cut them into quarters. Put the grated cauliflower into a pan together with the milk and simmer for 5 minutes. Drain and put to one side.

Heat the olive oil in a frying pan and fry the onion for 5 minutes. Add the salmon and cook for another 5 minutes. Then add the lemon juice, yoghurt and cumin and mix thoroughly.

Finally, combine the cauliflower with the salmon/vegetable mixture and top with the quartered eggs.

Full English Breakfast

An absolute classic, the English Breakfast has been maligned for years now due to it's fat content. However, it's now thought that the same fat may actually boost the metabolism for the rest of the day, and prime the body to burn fat more efficiently.

<u>Serves 1</u>   <u>Prep time 5m</u>   <u>Cook time 15m</u>

2 eggs
2 slices of bacon
2 sausages
1 large mushroom, sliced
2 slices of black pudding
1 tomato, cut in two
1 tsp of olive oil

Put the olive oil in a frying pan and fry the bacon, sausages and mushroom. When done, remove and place on a side dish. Next, fry the black pudding. Remove and place on the side dish. Do the same with the tomato.

Finally, fry the two eggs. Add to the side dish and, if necessary, give it a quick blast in the microwave to get it all nice and hot.

Almond Granola

This homemade granola is a healthier version of the shop-bought varieties, which are almost always much higher in sugar.

<u>Serves 10</u>   <u>Prep time 10m</u>   <u>Cook time 25m</u>

250g oats
40g flaked almonds
1 egg
2 tsp of honey
50g raisins
100g apricots, chopped
1 tsp olive oil

Preheat the oven to 150°C. Place the oats and almonds in a bowl and mix. In a separate bowl, beat the egg together with the honey until a frothy consistency has been achieved. Then add the oats and almonds and combine thoroughly.

Grease a baking sheet with the olive oil. Spread the mixture onto the baking sheet, place it in the oven and bake for about 15 minutes. Finally, add the raisins and apricots and bake for 10 more minutes

Low-Fat English Breakfast

In spite of the fact that the full English Breakfast is not now thought to be bad for you, there are still plenty of people who aren't so sure. This version is for them.

<u>Serves 1</u>   <u>Prep time 5m</u>   <u>Cook time 15m</u>

2 low-fat pork sausages
2 rashers of lean bacon, visible fat removed
1 large mushroom, quartered or sliced
1 small onion, cut into rings
1 tomato, halved
1 medium boiled potato, cubed
½ tin of baked beans
2 eggs

Grill the sausages for 5 minutes, turning frequently. Put them to one side when they are done and then grill the bacon.

Place the mushroom, onion, tomato and potato in a frying pan and fry until the mushroom, tomato and onion are softened and the potato is golden brown. Heat the beans in a small pan until ready.

Crack the eggs into a non-stick pan and cook to your liking. Assemble your breakfast on a large plate, adding brown sauce or tomato ketchup if desired.

Mushroom & Garlic Omelette

Omelettes make a fast and very filling meal, especially when they are served with salad.

<u>Serves 1</u>   <u>Prep time 5m</u>   <u>Cook time 10m</u>

3 eggs
100g mushrooms
1 tbsp olive oil
2 cloves garlic
1 tsp of mixed herbs
2 tbsp milk

Dice the mushrooms and garlic cloves as finely as you can. Then place in a mixing bowl with the rest of the ingredients and whisk to a frothy consistency.

Heat the olive oil in a small non-stick frying pan until it begins to bubble. Turn the heat down and then pour the mixture into the pan.

Cook the omelette until it is golden brown on the underside. Turn it over and cook for another thirty seconds or so.

Apple and Linseed Porridge

Start the day the right way with a nutrient-packed oaty breakfast - full of stomach-friendly fibre that is great for digestion.

<u>Serves 1</u>   <u>Prep time 5m</u>   <u>Cook time 6m</u>

50g rolled oats
1 apple
1 tsp ground nutmeg
250ml semi-skimmed milk
1 tbsp ground linseed
1 tsp honey

The first step is to peel and grate the apple. Then mix the grated apple with the nutmeg, oats and milk in a saucepan.

Bring to the boil then reduce the heat and cook for 5 minutes. Then stir in the ground linseed.

Pour into a breakfast bowl, add a drizzle of honey on top and your porridge is ready to eat.

Lunch Recipes

Carrot Kugel 28
Chicken Burritos 29
Thai Cauliflower Rice 30
Duck Stir Fry 31
Salmon & Avocado Burger 32
Mushroom Penne 33
Poached Plaice 34
Spicy Avocado Wraps 35
Ginger Garlic Salmon 36
Lentil Curry 37
Oriental Steamed Fish 39
Thai Chilli Satay 40
Five-Spice Pork 41
Pakistani Chickpeas 42
Salmon Fish Cakes 43
Quinoa Pilaf 44

Carrot Kugel

Kugel is a traditional Jewish dish. It's usually made with noodles and is sweet, but savoury versions can be made with potatoes or carrots. It makes an excellent light lunch or supper when served with salad, and can be eaten hot or cold.

<u>Serves 2</u>   <u>Prep time 10m</u>   <u>Cook time 25m</u>

1 egg
250g carrots
25g onion, grated
25g cheddar cheese, finely grated
25g cream cheese
1 clove garlic, crushed
1 tsp mustard
1 tsp sunflower oil

Put the egg, garlic, mustard, cream cheese and cheddar cheese in a bowl and mix well.

Grate the carrots and onion, add to the egg and cheese mixture, and beat vigorously until all the ingredients are thoroughly mixed.

Oil an oven-proof pie dish or tin. Then add the Kugel mixture and lightly press to ensure it's evenly spread in the tin. Bake in an oven preheated to 180°C for 20-25 minutes and then serve.

Chicken Burritos

These burritos are quick to prepare, filling and make a substantial lunch.

<u>Serves 2</u>   <u>Prep time 15m</u>   <u>Cook time 15m</u>

80g rice
2 tsp olive oil
1 onion
1 chicken breast, cut into chunks
1 pepper, de-seeded and chopped
1 clove garlic
1 tsp chilli powder
2 tortillas
1 tbsp cream cheese

First, put the rice on to cook in a pan.

In a separate pan, fry the onion, chicken and pepper in the olive oil for about 10 minutes.

Add the chilli powder and garlic and cook for another 2 minutes or so. When the rice is cooked, add it to the chicken and onion, and mix well.

Warm the tortillas and spread a layer of cream cheese on each one. Then add the chicken and rice mixture and roll up the tortillas, tucking in the ends, to form a neat parcel.

Thai Cauliflower Rice

This low calorie meal is perfect for a quick lunch. Rather than use carbohydrate-high rice though, the recipe uses grated cauliflower as a healthier substitute.

<u>Serves 2</u>   <u>Prep time 10m</u>   <u>Cook time 10m</u>

2 tsp olive oil
1 onion
1/2 pepper, de-seeded and chopped
70g pineapple, cut into small chunks
2 tbsp Thai green curry paste
1/2 cauliflower, grated
70g peas
100g can bamboo shoots, drained
100g prawns
150ml semi-skimmed milk

Heat the olive oil in a frying pan and fry the onion for 2 minutes. Stir in the pepper, pineapple and the green curry paste and cook for 3 more minutes.

Put the cauliflower in a pan with the milk and simmer it for five minutes. Then drain the milk and return the cauliflower to the pan.

Stir the peas, bamboo shoots and prawns into the 'cauliflower rice', then cook for 2 or 3 minutes until the prawns are hot and the peas tender. Then add the onion and pepper mixture, stir well and serve.

Duck Stir Fry

Duck meat is lean and full of flavour, unlike much of the chicken sold these days. This meal goes well with rice.

<u>Serves 2</u>   <u>Prep time 10m</u>   <u>Cook time 15m</u>

4 duck breasts
1 tsp Chinese Five Spice
300g pak choi (Chinese cabbage)
2 tbsp olive oil
2 peppers, de-seeded and sliced
150g sugar snap peas, sliced lengthways
3cm root ginger, finely chopped
1 red chilli, de-seeded and sliced
100g black bean sauce
1 tsp coriander

Roughly chop the pak choi – keep the stalk and leaf ends separate.

Heat half the oil in a frying pan and stir-fry the duck for five minutes. Put into a bowl and set aside. Heat the remaining oil and fry the peppers, sugar snap peas and pak choi stalks for a few minutes until they are soft. Add the ginger, pak choi leaves and chilli, and fry for a couple more minutes.

Return the duck to the pan together with the black bean sauce and 100ml of water. Heat through, sprinkle with the coriander and serve.

Salmon & Avocado Burger

A variation on the standard hamburger, the Salmon & Avocado Burger is not just healthier, it is considerably tastier.

<u>Serves 2</u>   <u>Prep time 5m</u>   <u>Cook time 10m</u>

2 spring onions, roughly chopped
1 handful of parsley
1 handful of rocket
250g salmon fillets
1/2 avocado, sliced
50g fresh breadcrumbs
1 tsp hot horseradish sauce
1 egg
1 tbsp olive oil

Using a food processor, mix the spring onions, parsley, avocado and salmon until finely chopped. Put the mixture into a large bowl and stir in the breadcrumbs, horseradish sauce, the egg and some seasoning.

Shape the mixture into 4 patties. Heat the olive oil in a large non-stick frying pan over a low-medium heat and then fry the patties for 5 minutes on either side, or until golden and cooked through.

Serve the burgers on a bed of rocket and a wedge of lemon or lime.

Mushroom Penne

Add protein to a vegan pasta dish by using a low-fat hummus in the sauce. With the mushrooms and low-carb pasta, you have a healthy and filling lunch.

<u>Serves 2</u>   <u>Prep time 20m</u>   <u>Cook time 15m</u>

200g chickpeas
1 tbsp lemon juice
1 garlic clove
1 tsp vegetable bouillon
2 tsp tahini
¼ tsp ground coriander
115g low-carb penne pasta
2 tsp olive oil
2 onions, halved and sliced
200g mushrooms, roughly chopped
1 handful of parsley

The first step is to put the pasta on to cook. Then make the hummus. Do this by tipping the chickpeas into a bowl with the lemon juice, garlic, bouillon, tahini and coriander. With a blender, mix to a wet paste.

Heat the oil in a frying pan and fry the onions and mushrooms. Drain the pasta and tip in the onions and mushrooms. Remove from the heat and mix in the houmous and parsley. Squeeze the lemon juice over and serve.

Poached Plaice

Fillets of poached plaice in fish stock, served on a bed of samphire, make a light and succulent lunch.

<u>Serves 2</u>   <u>Prep time 10m</u>   <u>Cook time 20m</u>

150g carrots, halved lengthways
6 spring onions, chopped
400g samphire
5g dill, roughly chopped, plus 4 sprigs to serve
1 vegetable stock cube, dissolved in 500ml water
2 plaice fillets
1 tsp cornflour, dissolved in 1 tbsp skimmed milk
1 tbsp Greek yogurt

Cook the carrots in a pan of water.

Put the spring onions, dill and samphire in a pan with the plaice on top. Pour in the vegetable stock and bring to the boil. Cover and simmer for 5 minutes.

When the fish is cooked, remove it from the pan. Then put the carrots, spring onions and samphire onto plates and place the fish on top.

Stir the cornflour into the boiling stock until thickened, then add the yogurt. Mix well, then pour over the fish. Sprinkle with pepper and serve with a wedge of lemon and a sprig of dill.

Spicy Avocado Wraps

A tasty, healthy, and extremely quick and easy meal to prepare.

<u>Serves 2</u>   <u>Prep time 5m</u>   <u>Cook time 8m</u>

150g of Quorn chicken-style pieces
1 avocado
1 pepper, de-seeded and chopped
½ tsp chilli powder
1 garlic clove, chopped
1 tbsp olive oil
2 tortilla wraps
1 handful of coriander, chopped
1 lime, juice of

Mix the chicken-style pieces with the lime juice, chilli powder and garlic. Then pile it all into a frying pan and fry in the olive oil for 2 or 3 minutes.

Add the chopped pepper and fry until the pepper is cooked.

Squash half the avocado meat on to each tortilla wrap and then add the chicken-style piece mix. Sprinkle the coriander over it all, roll up the tortilla wraps and you're ready to eat.

Ginger Garlic Salmon

Another extremely quick and easy lunch to prepare. I do, however, advise you not to eat salmon bought in supermarkets or labelled as 'Atlantic salmon'. They all come from fish farms and are exposed to pollutants such as dioxin and DDT, not to mention carcinogens. These chemicals can cause a range of health issues.

Alaskan salmon is what you want - it is actually illegal to farm Alaskan salmon.

<u>Serves 2</u>   <u>Prep time 5m</u>   <u>Cook time 10m</u>

2 salmon fillets
75g butter
1 tbsp soy sauce
1 clove garlic
3cm root ginger, finely chopped or grated
1 tsp brown sugar
1 lemon, juice of

Preheat the oven grill. Then grill the salmon for about five minutes on both sides.

Heat the butter in a small saucepan and then add the soy sauce, garlic, ginger, brown sugar and lemon juice. Cook until nice and hot.

When done, pour the ginger garlic butter over the cooked salmon and serve.

Lentil Curry

This tasty vegetarian curry is perfect for a quick and easy supper.

<u>Serves 4</u>   <u>Prep time 10m</u>   <u>Cook time 25m</u>

3 tbsp olive oil
1 onion, finely chopped
1 garlic clove, finely chopped
2cm root ginger, grated
2 tsp ground coriander
2 tsp ground cumin
1/2 tsp ground turmeric
75g red or yellow lentils
150ml vegetable stock
1 cauliflower, cut into small florets
1 large carrot, diced
400ml can coconut milk
75g green beans
1 tbsp lemon juice
Salt and pepper
1 sprig of fresh coriander

Heat 2 tablespoons of the olive oil in a large saucepan and gently cook the onion for 10 minutes, stirring frequently, until soft. Add the garlic, ginger, coriander, cumin and turmeric and cook for 2 more minutes, stirring continuously.

Cont'd

Stir in the lentils, then pour in the vegetable stock. Bring to the boil, then reduce the heat, cover and gently simmer for 10 minutes.

Meanwhile, heat the remaining olive oil in a frying pan and fry the cauliflower for 2–3 minutes until lightly browned. Then add it to the lentil mixture together with the carrot and coconut milk.

Bring the curry back to a gentle simmer and cook for a further 10 minutes or until the vegetables are tender. Stir in the beans and cook for 3–4 minutes.

Add the chopped coriander and lemon juice then season to taste with salt and pepper. Transfer the curry to a warmed serving dish and garnish it with a sprig of fresh coriander.

Oriental Steamed Fish

Steaming keeps in all the goodness and flavour, while the oriental flavours of chilli, ginger and lemon work brilliantly with white fish.

<u>Serves 2</u>   <u>Prep time 10m</u>   <u>Cook time 15m</u>

2 fish fillets
2cm root ginger, chopped
1 garlic clove, chopped
1 red chilli, finely chopped
1 lime, grated zest of
1 tbsp lime juice
1 pak choi, chopped
2 tbsp soy sauce

Place the fish fillets side by side on a large square of foil and then sprinkle the ginger, garlic, chilli and lime zest over them.

Drizzle the lime juice on top and then sprinkle the pieces of pak choi around and on top of the fish. Pour the soy sauce over everything and loosely seal the foil to make a package - make sure you leave space at the top for the steam to circulate as the fish cooks.

Steam for 15 minutes. If you haven't got a steamer, put the package on a heatproof plate over a pan of gently simmering water, cover with a lid and steam.

Thai Chilli Satay

This recipe uses Shirataki noodles, which are also known as 'miracle noodles', due to their very low carbohydrate content.

<u>Serves 4</u>　　　<u>Prep time 5m</u>　　　<u>Cook time 10m</u>

3 tbsp crunchy peanut butter
3 tbsp sweet chilli sauce
2 tbsp soy sauce
300g Shirataki noodles
1 tbsp olive oil
2cm root ginger, grated
300g pack mixed stir-fry vegetables
1 handful of basil leaves

Mix the peanut butter, chilli sauce, 100ml water and soy sauce to make a smooth satay sauce. Put the noodles in a bowl and pour boiling water over them. Stir gently to separate, then drain thoroughly.

Heat the oil in a frying pan or wok, then stir-fry the ginger and harder pieces of veg from the stir-fry mix, such as peppers, for 2 minutes. Add the noodles and the rest of the vegetables, then stir-fry over a high heat for 1-2 minutes until the vegetables are cooked.

Add the satay sauce to the pan and mix with the vegetables and noodles. Cook until hot then put on serving plates. Sprinkle with the basil leaves to finish.

Five-Spice Pork

Chinese 5 spice powder, with it's special blend of five classic spices, garlic and pepper, adds a delicious and distinctive flavour to this pork and vegetable stir fry.

<u>Serves 2</u>   <u>Prep time 20m</u>   <u>Cook time 15m</u>

200g pork fillet, cut into strips
15g egg noodles
1 tbsp olive oil
1 small onion, finely chopped
1 garlic clove, crushed
1 tbsp five-spice powder
150g sugar snap peas
1 pepper, de-seeded and thinly sliced
50ml hot vegetable stock

Cook the noodles in a saucepan of boiling water for five minutes. Drain and set aside. Then stir-fry the onion and garlic in the olive oil for one minute. Put the five-spice powder in next and continue frying for another minute.

Add the pork strips to the pan and stir-fry for three minutes. Next in are the sugar snap peas and the pepper - stir-fry for a further 2 minutes. Pour in the stock, stir well and bring to the boil.

Add the noodles to the pan, and stir and toss until all the ingredients are well combined. Serve.

Pakistani Chickpeas

Tender cooked chickpeas are simmered lightly with tomatoes, lemon juice and onions in a spicy blend of toasted cumin seeds and chilli powder.

<u>Serves 2</u>   <u>Prep time 10m</u>   <u>Cook time 20m</u>

1 onion, chopped
1 tomato, chopped
200g chickpeas
1 tbsp olive oil
1 tsp cumin seeds
1/2 tsp salt
1/2 tsp chilli powder
1 tbsp lemon juice

Heat the cumin seeds in the olive oil until they turn a dark shade of brown.

Add the salt and chilli powder, and mix well. Stir in the chopped tomato and when the juice begins to thicken, add the chickpeas and mix well.

Finally, add the onion and lemon juice. Cook until the onion is soft. Remove from heat and serve immediately.

While it's a fact that chickpeas have quite a high level of carbohydrates, when eaten in conjunction with healthy oils and vegetables, the carbs are released slowly and so don't cause a spike in blood sugar levels.

Salmon Fish Cakes

If you're after something that's a bit lighter than potato-packed fish cakes, try this simple oriental-style version.

<u>Serves 4</u>   <u>Prep time 20m</u>   <u>Cook time 10m</u>

4 salmon fillets, cut into chunks
2 tbsp Thai red curry paste
2cm root ginger, grated
1 tsp soy sauce
1 bunch coriander, chopped
1 tsp olive oil
1 lemon, cut into wedges
2 carrots
1 small cucumber
2 tbsp white wine vinegar
1 tsp caster sugar

Put the salmon into a food processor with the curry paste, ginger, soy sauce and chopped coriander. Pulse until roughly minced. Remove the mixture and shape it into four burger-size cakes.

Heat the oil in a frying pan then fry the cakes for 4-5 minutes on each side. Next, peel strips of carrot and cucumber into a bowl. Toss with the vinegar and sugar until the sugar has dissolved, then toss through the coriander leaves. Divide the salad between four plates. Serve with the fish cakes together with the lemon.

Quinoa Pilaf

This creamy pilaf combines fluffy, nutty-flavoured quinoa with a delicious cheese to give a most unusual flavour and texture.

<u>Serves 1</u>   <u>Prep time 10m</u>   <u>Cook time 30m</u>

4 tbsp quinoa
3 tbsp olive oil
2 tbsp raw sunflower seeds
2 cloves garlic, minced
50g spinach leaves
2 tsp lemon juice
25g grated hard cheese, such as cheddar

Bring a pot of lightly salted water to the boil. Add the quinoa and cook until it is soft. Drain and set aside.

Heat the olive oil in a frying pan, stir in the sunflower seeds and cook for about 2 minutes until lightly toasted. Stir in the garlic and cook for 2 more minutes.

Add the cooled quinoa and spinach leaves and stir until the quinoa is hot and the spinach has wilted.

Add the lemon juice and all but a pinch of the cheese. Stir until the cheese has melted. Serve sprinkled with the remaining cheese.

Dinner Recipes

Jollof Chicken Rice 46

Prawn Biryani 48

Chicken & Chorizo Jambalaya 50

Sausage Stew 51

Venison Stir-Fry 52

Tandoori Chicken 53

Creamy Courgette Lasagne................................... 54

Spicy Chicken & Broccoli Stir Fry 55

Pepper Ciambotta 56

Barbecue Pork Steaks 57

Chilli Casserole 58

Almond Nachos 59

Vegetable Paella 61

Chinese Braised Beef 63

Chicken And Leek Pie 65

Cauliflower Pizza 67

Beef Goulash 68

Nut Roast 70

Aubergine & Courgette Bake................................ 72

Mushroom Risotto 73

Fish Stew 74

Chicken Fajitas 76

Jollof Chicken Rice

A popular West African dish that's cooked in one pan and is ideal for a simple, quick and tasty dinner.

<u>Serves 4</u>   <u>Prep time 15m</u>   <u>Cook time 30m</u>

2 tsp olive oil
1 large onion, chopped
350g chicken breast, cut into chunks
1 red pepper, chopped
1 yellow pepper, chopped
400g dry Shirataki rice
2 garlic cloves, crushed
3 cm ginger, finely chopped
1 Scotch Bonnet chilli, chopped
2 tbsp tomato purée
1 chicken stock cube dissolved in 450ml water
400g can chopped tomatoes
100g okra, chopped into 2cm pieces
2 tbsp chopped coriander

Heat the oil in a large pan then add the onion and cook for 3-4 minutes until it's starting to brown.

Add the chicken chunks and cook for a further 3-4 minutes, stirring regularly to make sure the chicken cooks evenly.

Next into the pan is the red and yellow peppers. Carry on cooking for another 2 minutes before adding the

Cont'd

garlic, ginger, chilli and tomato puree. Mix thoroughly and then add the rice, chicken stock and tomatoes. Bring to the boil, reduce the heat, cover and simmer for 10 minutes or so.

Scatter the okra on top of the rice, replace the lid and simmer a further 5 minutes.

Now turn off the heat but don't remove the lid. Leave to stand for 5 minutes. Add the coriander, give it one last stir and serve.

Note: Shirataki rice and noodles are both made from the root of a plant called Konnyaku. As they are made from the soluble fibre of the plant, they are extremely low in calories.

Prawn Biryani

A fragrantly spiced pilaf-style dish that doesn't take much more effort than ringing for a take-away yet is far healthier. Grated cauliflower is used instead of rice.

<u>Serves 4</u>   <u>Prep time 15m</u>   <u>Cook time 15m</u>

400g can chopped tomatoes
300g baby leaf spinach, chopped
2 tbsp olive oil
1 onion, thinly sliced
1 red chilli, de-seeded and thinly sliced
1cm root ginger, finely chopped
1 tbsp ground cumin
1 tbsp ground coriander
1 tsp ground turmeric
½ tsp ground nutmeg
1/2 cauliflower, grated
1 pinch of sugar
225g peeled tiger prawns

Sieve the tomatoes over a heatproof measuring jug, place in a bowl and then set aside. Keep the sieved juice that's in the jug. Put a kettle of water on to boil.

Heat the oil in a large flame-proof casserole dish over a medium heat. Add the onion, chilli and ginger, and stir for 3 minutes.

Stir in the cumin, coriander, turmeric and nutmeg and

Cont'd

continue stirring until the onion is cooked.

Add the grated cauliflower and drained tomatoes to the casserole and stir to mix with the spices. Add enough boiling water to the reserved tomato juice to make up to 450ml. Stir this liquid and the sugar into the casserole, add a pinch of salt, then bring to the boil.

Reduce the heat to low, cover tightly and leave the 'cauliflower rice' to cook without lifting the lid for 10–12 minutes.

Then stir in the spinach in small batches, adding more as each addition wilts. When all the spinach has been added, lay the prawns on top, re-cover the casserole and turn the heat down to very low.

Cook for 2 minutes, then turn off the heat and leave to stand for 1 minute, without lifting the lid. By this time the spinach will have wilted further and the prawns will have cooked through. Gently fork together to combine the cauliflower rice, spinach and prawns and then serve immediately.

Chicken & Chorizo Jambalaya

A Cajun-inspired rice pot recipe with spicy Spanish sausage, sweet peppers and tomatoes. Low-carb dry Shirataki rice is used instead of normal rice.

<u>Serves 4</u>   <u>Prep time 10m</u>   <u>Cook time 35m</u>

2 chicken breasts, chopped
1 onion, chopped
1 red pepper, thinly sliced
250g dry Shirataki rice
400g can plum tomatoes
2 garlic cloves, crushed
1 tbsp olive oil
75g chorizo, sliced
1 tbsp Cajun seasoning
350ml chicken stock

Heat the oil in a large frying pan and cook the chicken for 5 minutes or so. Remove and set aside.

Add the onion and cook for 3-4 minutes until soft. Then add the pepper, garlic, chorizo and Cajun seasoning, and cook for another 5 minutes.

Cook the Shirataki rice by simmering it in a separate pan of water for 20 minutes. Then drain the water and add the rice, the chicken and the chicken stock to the pan containing the pepper, garlic, chorizo and Cajun

Sausage Stew

Sausages are a favourite food all over the world. This recipe presents them in a somewhat unusual way.

<u>Serves 4</u>　　　<u>Prep time 10m</u>　　　<u>Cook time 20m</u>

8 sausages
1 tsp olive oil
2 tsp dried oregano
2 garlic cloves, sliced
400g can chopped tomatoes
200ml beef stock
100g pitted black olives in brine
500g mushrooms, thickly sliced

Cut the sausages into meatball-size pieces. Then heat a large pan and fry the sausage pieces in the oil for about 5 minutes until browned all over.

Add the oregano and garlic, fry for 1 more minute, then add the tomatoes, stock, olives and mushrooms.

Simmer for 15 minutes until the sausages are cooked through and the sauce has thickened. Serve the sausage stew with mashed potato or pasta.

Venison Stir-Fry

Venison is a lovely, tasty meat. It also has half the calories and just one sixth of the amount of saturated fat found in beef. Give it a try with this delicious stir-fry.

<u>Serves 2</u>   <u>Prep time 15m</u>   <u>Cook time 10m</u>

2 tbsp sesame oil
8 cherry tomatoes
300g venison, cut into thin strips
1 small leek, cut into fine strips
1/2 pepper, finely sliced
1 tbsp soy sauce
3 tbsp sweet chilli dipping sauce
3 tbsp olive oil
Salt and pepper

Heat 1 tbsp of sesame oil in a pan and fry the tomatoes for two minutes. Add the venison, leek and pepper, and stir-fry for a further 5 minutes. Then add the soy sauce and cook for another 3 minutes. Season with salt and pepper to taste.

To make the dressing, mix the sweet chilli sauce, olive oil and 1 tbsp of sesame oil together in a small bowl.

To serve, place the venison stir fry on a serving platter and drizzle with the dressing.

Tandoori Chicken

This low-fat curried chicken is packed full of flavour. It's quick to cook and the marinade does all the work.

<u>Serves 4</u>   <u>Prep time 30m</u>   <u>Cook time 15m</u>

8 chicken thighs
1 red onion, finely chopped
1 lemon, juice of
2 tsp paprika
1 tsp olive oil

For the marinade:
300ml Greek yogurt
2cm root ginger, grated
2 garlic cloves, crushed
1/2 tsp garam masala
1/2 tsp ground cumin
¼ tsp turmeric

Mix the lemon juice with the paprika and red onion in a large shallow dish. Slash the chicken thighs then turn them in the juice and put to one side.

Mix the marinade and pour over the chicken. Cover and chill for at least one hour.

Place the chicken pieces onto a hot grill. Brush with a little olive oil and grill until lightly charred and completely cooked through. Serve.

Creamy Courgette Lasagne

Quick, easy to prepare and meat-free, this lasagne is ideal for vegetarians.

<u>Serves 4</u>   <u>Prep time 10m</u>   <u>Cook time 20m</u>

9 low-carb lasagne sheets
1 tbsp olive oil
1 onion, finely chopped
3 courgettes, finely chopped
2 garlic cloves, crushed
250g tub ricotta
50g cheddar cheese, grated
350g jar pasta tomato sauce

Pre-heat the oven to 220°C. Cook the lasagne sheets for about 5 minutes until soft. Rinse and then drizzle with a little oil to stop them sticking together.

In a frying pan, fry the onion in the olive oil. After 3 minutes, add the chopped courgette and garlic and keep frying until the courgette has softened. Stir in two thirds of both the ricotta and the cheddar cheese, then season to taste. Heat the tomato sauce until hot.

In a large baking dish, layer the ingredients starting with half the courgette mix, then pasta, then tomato sauce. Repeat, top with blobs of the remaining ricotta, then scatter the rest of the cheddar. Bake in the oven for about 10 minutes.

Spicy Chicken & Broccoli Stir Fry

Garlic, dried red chillies and chilli paste add some spice to chicken and broccoli.

Serves 4   Prep time 20m   Cook time 30m

275g broccoli florets
1 tbsp olive oil
2 chicken breast fillets cut into strips
1/2 bunch spring onions, sliced
4 cloves garlic, thinly sliced
1 tbsp hoisin sauce
1 tbsp chilli paste
1 tbsp light soy sauce
1/2 tsp ground ginger
1/4 tsp dried crushed chillies
4 tbsp chicken stock

Cook the broccoli in a steamer until it's tender but still firm. Heat the oil in a frying pan over a medium heat and stir-fry the chicken, spring onions and garlic until the chicken is cooked.

Add the hoisin sauce, chilli paste and soy sauce to the frying pan. Season with the ginger, chillies, salt and black pepper. Then stir in the chicken stock and simmer for about 2 minutes.

Finally, mix in the steamed broccoli until it's well coated with the sauce mixture. Serve.

Pepper Ciambotta

Ciambotta is a vegetable stew, the ingredients of which can vary according to what's on hand. It makes a delicious accompaniment to roasted chicken, fish or meat.

<u>Serves 4</u>   <u>Prep time 15m</u>   <u>Cook time 45m</u>

2 tbsp olive oil
1 large onion, chopped
2 small fennel bulbs
2 cloves of garlic
1 pepper, chopped
1 can tomatoes
2 medium courgettes, chopped
200g green beans, chopped
1 handful of basil leaves

Heat the olive oil and then add the onion and fennel. Cook for 15 minutes or until the vegetables are lightly browned and tender, stirring occasionally. Add the pepper and garlic, and cook for another 5-7 minutes.

Add the tomatoes with their juice, the courgettes, green beans and 1/2 teaspoon of salt. Raise the heat to medium-high, stirring and breaking up the tomatoes. Then lower the heat to medium-low, cover, and simmer for 2530 minutes or until all the vegetables are tender. Top with the basil and serve.

Barbecue Pork Steaks

Pork steaks marinated in garlic and lemon, cooked with apple and red onion. These can be barbecued, cooked in a griddle pan or grilled.

<u>Serves 4</u>   <u>Prep time 20m</u>   <u>Cook time 15m</u>

4 lean pork loin steaks
6 cloves garlic, crushed
1 lemon, juice of
2 apples
2 red onions
2 tsp balsamic vinegar

Put the pork, garlic and lemon juice in a food bag, seal it and then give it a good shake so the pork is thoroughly coated. Put it to one side. De-core the apples and cut them into 16 wedges. Slice the onions into rings leaving the skin on - this holds them together.

Put the apple wedges and slices of onion onto the BBQ, or griddle pan, and grill for about 10 minutes turning as necessary. When the onions are cooked, remove their skin and drizzle the vinegar onto them.

Cook the pork steaks for 3-5 minutes on each side, depending on thickness. When done, remove them from the barbecue and cover with foil. Leave to rest for 3-4 minutes, before serving with the onion and apple.

Chilli Casserole

Chilli casserole can be served by itself in bowls with grated cheese and sour cream. It can also be eaten with rice.

<u>Serves 4</u>   <u>Prep time 5m</u>   <u>Cook time 20m</u>

1 onion, sliced
500g mince meat
2 cloves garlic, crushed
1 pepper, diced
200g can tomatoes
2 tsp tomato paste
100g grated cheese
2 tsp ground cumin
2 tsp ground coriander
1 tsp chilli powder

Fry the onion and garlic until soft, add the mince and cook until all the meat has browned. Add the pepper and cook until it's soft.

Add all the other ingredients, stir and cook for about 5 minutes. Then pour into a baking dish. Sprinkle the grated cheese on top and cook at 180°C for 20 minutes.

Garnish with sour cream and a sprinkle of coriander, divide into four bowls and then serve.

Almond Nachos

Nachos are a very popular Mexican dish, an important ingredient of which is tortilla chips. Made with almond flour, the chips in this recipe are low-carb and very good for you.

<u>Serves 6</u>　　　<u>Prep time 20m</u>　　　<u>Cook time 20m</u>

Tortilla Chips
170g mozzarella cheese, grated
85g almond flour
2 tbsp cream cheese
1 egg
1 tsp cumin
1 tsp coriander
1 tsp chilli powder
2 tsp olive oil

Nacho Meat Sauce
1 onion, diced
500g minced meat
400g can tomatoes, chopped
1 tbsp tomato paste

To make the meat sauce, fry the diced onion in the olive oil and then add and cook the minced meat for about 5 minutes. Add the tomatoes and tomato paste. Stir, then leave it to simmer over a low heat for 15 minutes whilst you make the tortilla chips and toppings.

Cont'd

To make the tortilla chips, mix the grated cheese and almond flour in a bowl. Then add the cream cheese and microwave on HIGH for one minute.

Stir then microwave on HIGH for another 30 seconds. Remove and stir again. Add the egg and the spices. Mix thoroughly to a pastry-like consistency.

Place the 'pastry' between 2 sheets of baking paper and roll it into a thin rectangle. Remove the top piece of baking paper and slide the baking paper with the pastry onto a baking tray and bake at 220C for 12-15 minutes, or until brown on the top. Flip the pastry over and brown the other side.

Once cooked, remove the pastry from the oven and cut it into tortilla chip triangle shapes. Bake again at 220°C for 3-5 minutes.

To put it all together, place a handful of the tortilla chips on a plate. Ladle the meat sauce over the chips and then add the grated cheese, which will melt on the hot meat sauce. Serve with a side salad if desired.

Vegetable Paella

Perfect for vegetarians, but great for meat-eaters too, this hearty rice dish made with low-carb dry Shirataki rice is wonderfully rich and satisfying.

<u>Serves 4</u>   <u>Prep time 15m</u>   <u>Cook time 30m</u>

3 tbsp olive oil
1 onion, chopped
2 garlic cloves, crushed
2 courgettes, chopped
2 carrots, peeled and chopped
250g dry Shirataki rice
200g chopped tomatoes
1 tsp turmeric
1 tsp paprika
800ml vegetable stock
100g French beans, chopped
100g frozen peas
2 tbsp parsley, chopped

Heat the oil in a frying pan. Add the onion and garlic, and cook for 2 minutes without letting them brown. Add the courgettes, carrots and vegetable stock. Cook for another 5 minutes or so over a high heat, stirring constantly. When done, put to one side.

Next, cook the Shirataki rice by simmering it in water for 20 minutes. Drain the water.

Cont'd

When the rice is ready, add it to the pan that contains the vegetables. Give it all a good stir and then add the tomatoes with their juice, and the turmeric and paprika.

Now cook the beans and peas in boiling water for 5 minutes. Drain and add both to the rice and vegetables.

Cook for a couple of minutes to make sure everything is good and hot, sprinkle the parsley on top and then serve.

Chinese Braised Beef

The perfect dinner when you fancy something hearty and warming. It comes with some exotic flavours as well that are sure to intrigue you.

<u>Serves 4</u>   <u>Prep time 10m</u>   <u>Cook time 120m</u>

2 tbsp olive oil
1 glass red wine
3 cloves of garlic, thinly sliced
3cm piece of root ginger, grated
1 bunch of spring onions, sliced
1 red chilli, de-seeded and sliced
1½ kg braising beef, cut into large chunks
2 tbsp plain flour
1 tsp Chinese five-spice powder
2 tbsp dark soy sauce
300ml beef stock

Heat the olive oil in a large frying pan and fry the garlic, ginger, onions and chilli for 3 minutes until soft. Put on a plate and place to one side.

Toss the beef in the flour then put it in the frying pan in batches as necessary. Cook each batch for about 5 minutes until brown.

Add the five-spice powder to the pan together with the onion, garlic, ginger and chilli mixture and fry it for 2

Cont'd

minutes or so. Lastly, splash in the wine.

Transfer everything to a casserole dish and add the soy sauce and beef stock. Place the cover on the casserole dish and put it in an oven pre-heated to 150ºC .

Cook for 2 hours stirring the meat halfway through. The meat should be very soft, and any sinewy bits should have melted. It will now be ready to eat.

Basmati rice is the perfect complement to Chinese braised beef.

Chicken And Leek Pie

Low in carbohydrates thanks to the almond flour, this chicken and leek pie is the basis of a dinner that the whole family will enjoy.

<u>Serves 6</u>   <u>Prep time 20m</u>   <u>Cook time 30m</u>

Pie Crust
55g butter
100g almond meal flour
1/2 tsp salt
1 egg
1 tbsp psyllium husk
2 tbsp coconut flour

Pie Filling
55g butter
1 leek, chopped
800g chicken, diced
200g cream cheese
200g cheddar cheese, grated
4 eggs
Salt and pepper

To make the crust, melt the butter and then add it to a bowl together with the almond flour and salt. Mix well. Then add the egg, psyllium husk and coconut flour, and mix again until a dough is formed.

Cont'd

Press the dough into a greased and lined pie dish with deep sides, or a casserole dish. Put it in the oven and bake at 180°C for 10 minutes or until just starting to brown. Remove from the oven.

To make the pie filling, melt the butter in a pan and add the chopped leek. Cook for 5 minutes, stirring occasionally, until it's cooked.

Remove the leek from the pan and put it to one side. Using the same pan, now cook the diced chicken.

When the chicken is cooked, reduce the heat, add the cream cheese and stir until it melts. Cook gently for a further 3-5 minutes.

Now put all the pie filling ingredients into a large bowl and mix them thoroughly. Then add the eggs and mix again.

Pour the pie filling into the cooked pie crust, place it in the oven and bake at 180°C for about 20 minutes until golden on top.

Cauliflower Pizza

This dish is a sneaky way to get more veggies into your children. The cheese masks the 'cauliflower' flavour.

<u>Serves 4</u>   <u>Prep time 20m</u>   <u>Cook time 20m</u>

1 medium cauliflower, finely chopped
1 egg
100g grated mozzarella cheese
1 tbsp each of rosemary and oregano
Salt and pepper

Cut the cauliflower into small pieces, put them in a food processor and blitz until quite fine. Then steam them until they are soft, or microwave for 5 minutes.

Place the cauliflower onto a clean tea towel and twist to remove all the liquid - if not enough liquid is removed, the pizza base won't crisp. Put the drained cauliflower in a large mixing bowl and add the egg, seasoning, herbs and grated cheese. Mix until a dough is formed.

Prepare a baking tray lined with a sheet of baking paper. Place the ball of 'cauliflower dough' onto the baking sheet and press it into a round pizza shape.

Brush the top with some olive oil to help it crisp, then bake at 180°C for 15 minutes or until golden. Finally, add the desired toppings, cover with more cheese and cook until the cheese is melted and bubbling. Then serve.

Beef Goulash

A fancy way of dressing up stewing beef. It's spicy but not mouth-burningly so!

<u>Serves 6</u>   <u>Prep time 20m</u>   <u>Cook time 150m</u>

1kg braising steak
1 tbsp olive oil
2 onions, sliced
4 garlic cloves, crushed
2 tbsp paprika
1 beef stock cube
500ml cold water
400g can chopped tomatoes
2 tbsp tomato purée
2 bay leaves
2 peppers
Salt and pepper

Preheat the oven to 170°C. Cut the meat into 5cm chunks and season with salt and pepper.

Heat the olive oil in a large flame-proof casserole dish and then add the meat and fry until it's nicely browned.

Next, put the onions in the dish and cook with the meat for 5 minutes until they are soft. Add the crushed garlic and cook for a further minute, stirring regularly.

Sprinkle the paprika over the meat and crumble the

Cont'd

beef stock cube on top. Then add the water, tomatoes, tomato purée and bay leaves. Stir well and bring to a simmer. Then put the lid on the dish and transfer it to the oven.

While the meat is cooking, remove the core and seeds from the peppers and cut them into small chunks.

After one and a half hours, remove the dish from the oven. Stir in the peppers, put the lid back on and place the goulash back in the oven for a further hour or until the beef is tender. Then serve.

Nut Roast

An extremely satiating vegetarian loaf packed with nuts, fruit, spices and vegetables that is just perfect for an evening meal.

Serves 4   **Prep time 15m**   **Cook time 60m**

100g butternut squash
2 tbsp olive oil
1 onion, finely chopped
1 pepper, finely chopped
2 cloves garlic, crushed
150g mixed unsalted nuts
2 eggs
150g ground almonds
200g cooked chestnuts, finely chopped
2 tbsp water
1 tsp ground nutmeg
250g spinach
25g dried cranberries

First, cook the spinach. To do this, heat 1 tablespoon of olive oil in a pan and then start adding the spinach, a handful at a time. As each handful wilts, add another. Cook for a couple of minutes, stirring the spinach constantly. When done, put to one side.

De-seed the butternut squash and cut it into chunks. Place the chunks in a pan of boiling water and boil

Cont'd

until tender. Then mash them and put to one side.

Next, heat the remaining olive oil in a pan and add the onion, stirring regularly. When it's starting to brown, add the pepper and cook for about 5 minutes. Add the garlic, mix, remove from the heat and allow to cool.

Divide the nuts into 3 piles. Put one pile aside, roughly chop the second pile and finely chop the third pile.

Add the eggs to a bowl with the ground almonds, onion, pepper, finely chopped and roughly chopped nuts, the chestnuts, water and nutmeg. Mix thoroughly.

Rub olive oil around a 1lb loaf tin and line it with greaseproof paper. Then take two-thirds of the egg mixture and press it around the tin to line it, leaving room in the centre for the filling.

Add the butternut squash followed by a layer of spinach in the centre. Sprinkle the cranberries on top. Next, add the rest of the egg mixture to create a lid and sprinkle with the reserved whole nuts, pressing them gently into the topping.

Cover with a piece of foil and place the loaf in another, larger, oven dish. Fill it with water to half way up the loaf tin. Cook in the oven for 30 minutes at 170°C, then remove the foil and cook for another 10 minutes. Remove from the oven, turn out onto a plate and serve.

Aubergine & Courgette Bake

This recipe is a much healthier version of a classic Italian dish.

<u>Serves 4</u>   <u>Prep time 30m</u>   <u>Cook time 50m</u>

2 large aubergines, cut into chunks
2 courgettes, cut into strips
1 tbsp olive oil
1 onion, finely chopped
1 red pepper, finely chopped
2 cloves garlic, crushed
1 tsp dried oregano
400g can chopped tomatoes
50g parmesan cheese, finely grated
120g mozzarella cheese, thinly sliced

Grill the aubergines and courgettes until they are browned on each side. Next, heat the olive oil in a pan and fry the onion. Then add the red pepper, stirring constantly for 5 minutes. Mix in the garlic, oregano and tomatoes, and allow to simmer for 5 minutes.

Add some of the sauce to an oven-proof dish and put some of the aubergine and courgette slices on top. Then add more sauce and sprinkle with parmesan cheese. Repeat to create layers and top the final layer with the slices of mozzarella cheese. Place the dish in the oven and bake for 30–40 minutes at 180°C.

Mushroom Risotto

A creamy risotto made with barley rather than rice and topped with a variety of mushrooms.

<u>Serves 4</u>   <u>Prep time 15m</u>   <u>Cook time 40m</u>

2 tsp olive oil
400g mixed mushrooms, sliced
1 onion, chopped
1 pepper, chopped
250g pearl barley
2 cloves of garlic, crushed
1 tsp dried oregano
1 stock cube in 700ml boiling water
1 tbsp chopped basil
4 tbsp cream

Heat the olive oil in a pan and fry the onion. Add the pepper and garlic and cook for 2 minutes, then add the mixed mushrooms and cook for 2-3 minutes more.

Put a handful of mushrooms aside to garnish the dish.

Stir in the barley, add the stock and oregano, and mix well. Bring to the boil, then turn down the heat and simmer until the liquid is absorbed. The barley should be cooked but still firm.

Stir in the cream and the basil, scatter the reserved mushrooms on top to garnish and serve.

Fish Stew

A hearty Mediterranean seafood dinner, packed with vegetables and garlic.

<u>Serves 4</u>   <u>Prep time 15m</u>   <u>Cook time 20m</u>

1 carrot, diced
1 fish stock cube in 600ml of water
1/2 bulb fennel, sliced
1 pepper, sliced
1 leek, chopped
1 tsp turmeric
2 cloves garlic, crushed
2 tsp olive oil
4 x fish fillets, cut in half to give 8 pieces
150g king prawns
150g mussel meat
2 tomatoes, chopped
1 tbsp finely chopped parsley

Put the water in a pan with the stock cube, bring to the boil, then turn down the heat. Cover and simmer for 5 minutes. Then add the carrot, fennel, pepper, leek, turmeric and garlic. Mix thoroughly, then cover and simmer for a further 5 minutes.

Next, put 1 tsp of olive oil in a frying pan over a medium heat. When the pan is hot, add 4 pieces of fish and cook for 2-3 minutes. Turn them over and cook

Cont'd

for another 1-2 minutes. Place on a hot plate and cook the remaining fish fillets with the second teaspoon of olive oil.

Add the mussels and prawns to the vegetables and stock, bring to the boil and cook for 2 minutes.

Put the vegetables, prawns, mussels and broth in four bowls. Place the fish fillets on top, sprinkle with parsley, chopped tomato and a sprinkle of black pepper. Serve.

Chicken Fajitas

These smokey fajitas combine the best of Mexican cuisine with the rich taste of the American deep south.

Serves 4   Prep time 10m   Cook time 40m

1 tbsp Worcestershire sauce
1 tbsp soy sauce
1 tsp chilli powder
1 clove garlic, minced
1 tsp hot pepper sauce
500g chicken thighs, cut into strips
1 tbsp olive oil
1 onion, sliced
1 green pepper, sliced
1/2 lemon, juice of
4 tortillas

In a medium bowl, combine the Worcestershire sauce, soy sauce, chilli powder, garlic and pepper sauce. Add the chicken strips and turn several times to coat them thoroughly. Then leave them to marinate for 30 minutes.

Heat the olive oil in a large frying pan and add the chicken strips to the pan. Cook for 5 minutes. Add the onion and green pepper and cook for another 3 minutes. Remove from the heat and sprinkle with lemon juice. Spread the chicken, onion and green pepper mix onto the tortillas, roll them up and serve.

Salad Recipes

Greek Salad 78
Couscous Salad 79
Quinoa Salad 80
Thai Chicken Salad 81
Lemon and Feta Salad... 82
Squid and Pepper Salad 83
Vietnamese Beef Salad 84
Fire Salad 85
Indian Summer Salad 86
Avocado and Sunflower Salad 87
Sausage Salad 88

Greek Salad

In this classic Greek salad recipe, tomatoes, red onion and cucumbers are dressed with olive oil and finished with crumbled feta cheese.

Serves 4   **Prep time 10m**   **Cook time 0m**

3 tomatoes, cut into wedges
2 cucumbers, sliced
1 red onion, thinly sliced
4 tbsp olive oil
1 1/2 tsp dried oregano
200g feta cheese, crumbled
50g olives, pitted
Salt and pepper

In a salad bowl, mix the tomatoes, cucumber and onion. Sprinkle the mixture with salt and let it sit for a few minutes so that the salt can draw out the natural juices from the tomato and cucumber.

Drizzle with olive oil and sprinkle with oregano and pepper to taste. Finish by covering the salad with feta cheese and olives. Serve.

Couscous Salad

This quick and easy to prepare salad is the ideal way to use up odds and ends left over from other meals.

<u>Serves 6</u>   <u>Prep time 10m</u>   <u>Cook time 40m</u>

180g dried couscous
1 tsp vegetable stock granules
2 tomatoes, finely chopped
2cm of cucumber, finely chopped
4 spring onions, chopped
1/2 can sweetcorn, drained
2 tbsp fresh mint, chopped
1 tbsp lemon balm, chopped
1 tbsp lemon juice
1 tbsp olive oil
Salt and pepper

Prepare the couscous by placing it and the vegetable stock granules in a large bowl and covering with boiling water so that all the couscous is covered. Place a clean dry tea towel over the bowl and allow the steam to cook the couscous. After 10 minutes, fork it through to loosen the grains.

When the couscous is cool, add the other ingredients and mix well. Place in the fridge to cool for 30 minutes while all the herbs and mint flavour are absorbed by the couscous. Serve.

Quinoa Salad

A quinoa salad that's perfect for picnics, barbecues or packed lunches.

Serves 6   **Prep time 10m**   **Cook time 15m**

170g quinoa, rinsed
100g cherry tomatoes, halved
55g black olives, pitted and sliced
125g feta cheese, crumbled
4 tbsp roasted sunflower seeds
1 onion, finely chopped
4 tbsp fresh parsley, chopped
3 tbsp olive oil
3 tbsp lemon juice
1 tsp Dijon mustard
2cm root garlic, finely chopped

In a bowl, mix the tomatoes and onion and then put to one side. Next, in a medium saucepan, mix the quinoa with water and bring it to the boil. Let it simmer for 15 minutes before taking it off the heat to cool.

When it has, put it in a bowl together with the tomato and onion mix, the olives, feta cheese, sunflower seeds, and parsley. Toss to combine. In a separate bowl, whisk the olive oil, lemon juice, Dijon mustard and garlic to make a dressing. Pour the lemon dressing over the quinoa salad and toss. Then serve.

Thai Chicken Salad

The hot spiciness of this salad works well with the vegetables, creating a good balance of flavour and heat.

<u>Serves 6</u>   <u>Prep time 10m</u>   <u>Cook time 10m</u>

4 lime leaves
2 red chilli
3 garlic cloves
2cm root ginger
4 chicken breasts
1 tbsp olive oil, 1 tbsp sesame oil
1 tsp chilli powder
50ml fish sauce
3 tbsp lime juice
3 baby gem lettuces, leaves separated
1 cucumber, de-seeded and cut into strips
200g bean sprouts

Blitz the lime leaves, chillies, garlic and ginger in a blender until very finely chopped. Then mince the chicken breasts into tiny pieces. Heat both oils in a pan and then add the lime and chilli mixture. Stir-fry for 1 minute and then add the minced chicken and chilli powder. Stir-fry for 4 minutes more before adding the fish sauce. Cook for another 5 minutes.

Remove from the heat and pour the lime juice over the chicken. Serve with the lettuce, cucumber and bean sprouts.

Lemon and Feta Salad

A fresh and tasty salad that could have been designed for a summer's day. The pine nuts give it a deliciously crunchy texture.

<u>Serves 4</u>   <u>Prep time 10m</u>   <u>Cook time 5m</u>

250g fresh spinach
1 tbsp pine nuts
30g feta cheese
1 lemon, grated zest and juice of
1 tbsp olive oil
Black pepper

Wash the spinach, add it to a pan with a lid, and cook for 2-3 minutes. Drain off all the excess water and allow to it cool.

Cook the pine nuts in a dry pan and stir regularly for 1-2 minutes until they are just starting to brown. Then put to one side.

Spread the spinach on a plate and then crumble the feta cheese over it. Scatter the roasted pine nuts on top.

Finally, sprinkle the lemon zest over the dish and drizzle with the lemon juice and olive oil. Season with the black pepper and serve.

Squid and Pepper Salad

Found in every ocean, squid is one of the most widely available seafoods in the world, and is also one of the cheapest.

<u>Serves 6</u>   <u>Prep time 10m</u>   <u>Cook time 5m</u>

4 red peppers, *thinly sliced*
2 x 400g can chickpeas, *rinsed and drained*
1 bunch parsley, *roughly chopped*
1 red chilli, *de-seeded and chopped*
2 garlic cloves, *finely chopped*
4 tbsp olive oil
600g squid, *sliced into rings*
1 lemon, *zest and juice of*
Salt and pepper

Cook the peppers under the grill. Then put them in a large bowl together with the chickpeas, parsley, chilli and garlic. Mix thoroughly and put to one side.

Heat one tablespoon of olive oil in a frying pan and add the squid. Stir-fry it until cooked.

Then put the squid into the bowl that contains the peppers and other ingredients. Season everything with salt and pepper and then dress with the remaining oil, lemon juice and lemon zest. Serve.

Vietnamese Beef Salad

A light, filling and very healthy salad with tender beef and plenty of vegetables.

<u>Serves 6</u>   <u>Prep time 5m</u>   <u>Cook time 12m</u>

350g lean beef, cut into strips
1/2 tsp chilli flakes
2 cloves garlic, crushed
4cm root ginger, finely chopped
1 pepper, sliced
150g sweetcorn
300g bean sprouts
6 spring onions, finely chopped
1 tbsp olive oil
1/2 cucumber, finely chopped
1 lime, juice of
2 tsp soy sauce

Put the olive oil and the beef in a pan and cook for 4–5 minutes. Stir in the chilli flakes, garlic and ginger. Add the pepper, stir-frying for 2–3 minutes, followed by the baby sweetcorn. Stir-fry for 1 more minute. Add the bean sprouts and spring onions and fry for 2 minutes. Then remove from the heat and allow to cool.

Make the dressing by mixing the cucumber, lime juice and soy sauce in a bowl. Then add the cooled beef mixture, mix thoroughly and serve.

Fire Salad

Fajita seasoning makes this chicken salad a seriously HOT affair! It's also seriously high in nutrients.

<u>Serves 6</u>   <u>Prep time 5m</u>   <u>Cook time 20m</u>

2 chicken breast fillets
1 35g packet of Old El Paso Fajita Spice Mix
1 tbsp olive oil
1 400g can black beans, rinsed and drained
300g sweetcorn
100g salsa
300g mixed salad greens
1 onion, chopped
1 tomato, chopped

Coat the chicken with half of the fajita spice mix. Then heat the olive oil in a frying pan and cook the chicken for 8 minutes on each side. Cut it into strips and put them to one side.

In a saucepan, mix the beans, sweetcorn, salsa and the other half of the fajita seasoning. Heat over a medium heat until warm.

Then mix the salad greens, onion and tomato in a bowl and top with the chicken. Finally, dress it all with the bean and corn mixture.

Indian Summer Salad

Packed with antioxidants, this super-healthy, colourful salad counts as one of your 5-a-day.

<u>Serves 6</u>	<u>Prep time 20m</u>	<u>Cook time 0m</u>

3 carrots
1 bunch radishes
2 courgettes
1 small red onion
1 handful mint leaves, chopped
1 tbsp white wine vinegar
1 tsp Dijon mustard
1 tbsp mayonnaise
2 tbsp olive oil
Salt and pepper

Grate the three carrots into a bowl. Then thinly slice the radishes and courgettes and finely chop the onion. Mix all the vegetables together in the bowl with the mint leaves.

Make the dressing by putting the vinegar, mustard and mayonnaise in a bowl and whisking to a smooth creamy consistency. Then gradually whisk in the olive oil.

Add salt and pepper to taste and then drizzle the dressing over the salad.

Avocado and Sunflower Salad

A favourite summer salad! The sunflower seeds add texture and are also very nutritious.

<u>Serves 4</u>   <u>Prep time 15m</u>   <u>Cook time 0m</u>

1 tbsp red wine vinegar
1 tbsp balsamic vinegar
1 clove garlic, minced
1 tbsp mayonnaise
2 heads little gem lettuce
50g sunflower seeds
2 avocados - de-stoned and sliced
6 tbsp olive oil
Salt and pepper

Whisk the olive oil, red wine vinegar, balsamic vinegar, garlic and mayonnaise together to make the dressing. Season with salt and pepper to taste.

In a salad bowl, combine the lettuce and sunflower seeds. Toss with enough dressing to coat the salad thoroughly. Top with sliced avocado and serve.

Sausage Salad

A classic winter salad topped off with tasty sausage and onion.

Serves 4   Prep time 5m   Cook time 8m

1 tbsp olive oil
400g sausages
1 red onion, diced
1 tbsp mustard
1 tsp light muscovado sugar
16 cherry tomatoes
2 little gem lettuces
1 small avocado, de-stoned and diced
1/2 cucumber, diced
1 tbsp red wine vinegar

Heat the olive oil in a frying pan. Cut the sausages into chunks and add them to the pan together with the onion. Stir-fry for 2 minutes and then add the mustard, muscovado sugar and tomatoes. Fry for about 5 minutes, stirring, until the mixture is coated in the sweet mustard glaze.

Separate the lettuces into leaves and mix them with the avocado and cucumber. Then put the mixture onto a platter, ladle the hot sausage mixture on top and serve.

Soups

Lentil & Bacon Soup 90
Chickpea Soup 91
Chilli Bean Soup 92
Bulgar Mushroom Soup 93
Minestrone Soup... 95
Chicken Soup 96
Oriental Pumpkin Soup 97
Peanut Soup 98
Cauliflower Cheese Soup 99
Oriental Prawn Soup 100

Lentil & Bacon Soup

A warming soup for the colder weather. Easy to prepare and extremely tasty.

<u>Serves 4</u>	<u>Prep time 10m</u>	<u>Cook time 50m</u>

1 tbsp olive oil
4 rashers smoked back bacon, diced
1 large onion, chopped
3 sticks celery, chopped
2 carrots, chopped
110g split red lentils
1.2 ltr water
1 tsp dried parsley
Salt and pepper

In a large saucepan, heat the olive oil and then fry the chopped bacon until done. Add the onion and fry for a further 2 minutes. Then add the celery, carrots, parsley and lentils and cook for a further minute.

Pour in the water and bring to the boil. Turn down the heat and simmer, covered, for 35-40 minutes, stirring occasionally to prevent sticking.

The soup can be served as it is (chunky) or liquidised with a hand blender.

Chickpea Soup

Come home to a bowl of this filling, low-fat soup. It's perfect for vegetarians as well.

<u>Serves 4</u>   <u>Prep time 10m</u>   <u>Cook time 25m</u>

1 tbsp olive oil
1 onion, chopped
2 celery sticks, chopped
2 tsp ground cumin
500ml vegetable stock
400g can chopped plum tomatoes
400g can chickpeas, rinsed and drained
100g broad beans
1/2 lemon, zest and juice of
1 handful coriander or parsley, chopped
1 pinch black pepper

Heat the oil in a large saucepan, then fry the onion and celery for 10 minutes until softened, stirring frequently. Add the cumin and fry for another minute.

Next, add the vegetable stock, tomatoes and chickpeas, plus a good pinch of black pepper. Simmer for 8 minutes and then add the broad beans and lemon juice. Cook for a further 2 minutes.

Season to taste, top with a sprinkling of lemon zest and chopped coriander or parsley and serve.

Chilli Bean Soup

A rich Mexican-style tomato and bean soup that makes a hearty winter supper.

<u>Serves 4</u>   <u>Prep time 5m</u>   <u>Cook time 30ms</u>

1 tbsp olive oil
1 large onion, chopped
2 cloves garlic, crushed
2 red chillies, finely chopped
1 tsp ground cumin
1 tsp ground cinnamon
2 400g cans kidney beans, drained and rinsed
1 400g can chopped tomatoes
1.2 ltr vegetable stock

Heat the oil in a saucepan, add the onion, garlic and chillies and fry for 2-3 minutes. Add the cumin and cinnamon and continue to fry for a further minute.

Then add the kidney beans, the chopped tomatoes and the vegetable stock to the pan. Bring to the boil, cover and let it simmer for 20 minutes.

Transfer the soup to a food processor, or blender, and blitz it to a smooth liquid. Finally, return it to the pan and heat until hot.

Bulgar Mushroom Soup

This soup from Eastern Europe is primarily a mushroom soup but it gets a lot of flavour from the other ingredients.

<u>Serves 6</u>   <u>Prep time 10m</u>   <u>Cook time 50m</u>

50g unsalted butter
1 onion, chopped
2 large mushrooms, chopped
2 tsp dried dill
1 tbsp paprika
1 tbsp soy sauce
500ml chicken stock
250ml milk
3 tbsp plain flour
1 tsp salt
Black pepper
2 tsp lemon juice
4 tbsp chopped parsley
125ml sour cream

Melt the butter in a large pot over a medium heat. Cook the onions in the butter for 5 minutes.

Add the mushrooms and cook for 5 more minutes.

Stir in the dill, paprika, soy sauce and chicken stock. Then reduce the heat to low, cover the pot and allow it

Cont'd

to simmer for 15 minutes.

In a bowl, whisk the milk and flour together and then pour the mix into the soup. Stir well, cover and simmer for another 15 minutes.

Finally, add the salt, black pepper, lemon juice, parsley and sour cream. Mix thoroughly, heat up for a couple of minutes and then serve.

Minestrone Soup

The perfect solution to a cold night in? A warming bowl of this chunky and delicious soup.

<u>Serves 4</u>   <u>Prep time 5m</u>   <u>Cook time 20m</u>

3 carrots, chopped
1 onion, chopped
4 celery sticks, chopped
1 tbsp olive oil
2 garlic cloves, crushed
2 potatoes, diced
2 tbsp tomato purée
2 ltr vegetable stock
400g can tomatoes, chopped
1/2 head cabbage, shredded

In a food processor, blitz the carrots, onion and celery into small pieces. Heat the oil in a pan, add the processed vegetables, garlic and potatoes, and then cook over a high heat for 5 minutes until everything is soft.

Stir in the tomato purée, vegetable stock and tomatoes. Bring to the boil, then turn down the heat and simmer, covered, for 10 minutes.

Finally, add the cabbage and simmer for another 2 minutes. Season to taste and serve.

Chicken Soup

This delicious and easy-to-prepare chicken soup will give your local Chinese take-away a run for its money.

Serves 4   **Prep time 10m**   **Cook time 40m**

800ml chicken stock
400g sweetcorn
100g chicken meat, cooked and shredded
1/2 tsp pepper
2 tbsp cornflour
125ml water
1 tbsp sesame oil
1 handful spring onions, chopped

Put the chicken stock, sweetcorn and chicken in a pan and bring to the boil. Then reduce the heat and add the pepper. Return to the boil.

In a bowl, mix the cornflour with the water. Add this mixture to the boiling soup and stir thoroughly until well mixed.

Season the soup with sesame oil, adding a few drops at a time. Now let the soup simmer on a low heat for 30 minutes.

When it is ready, garnish it with the chopped spring onions and serve.

Oriental Pumpkin Soup

Flavours of the mysterious East give this seasonal soup an added twist.

Serves 6   Prep time 10m   Cook time 45m

1kg pumpkin, chopped
4 tsp olive oil
1 onion, sliced
1 tbsp grated ginger
3 tbsp Thai red curry paste
400ml coconut milk
850ml vegetable stock
1 tsp lime juice
1 tsp sugar
1 red chilli, sliced

Heat the oven to 200°C. Put the pumpkin in a roasting tin and mix with half the oil, half the lime juice and the sugar. Roast for 30 minutes until it's tender.

In a pan, fry the onion and ginger in the remaining oil for 2-3 minutes until soft. Then add the curry paste, the roasted pumpkin, all but 3 tbsp of the coconut milk and the stock. Bring to a simmer and leave it for 5 minutes.

Then, whisk the soup with a hand blender until it is smooth. Season it with salt and pepper and the remaining lime juice. Serve drizzled with the reminder of the coconut milk and the chilli slices.

Peanut Soup

A hearty soup which gets its delicious flavour and lovely colour from a combination of red peppers, tomatoes, peanut butter, chilli pepper and brown rice.

<u>Serves 6</u>   <u>Prep time 5m</u>   <u>Cook time 65m</u>

2 tbsp olive oil
2 small onions, chopped
2 red peppers, chopped
4 cloves garlic, minced
700g jar passata
2 ltr vegetable stock
1/2 tsp black pepper
1/2 tsp chilli powder
200g crunchy peanut butter
85g uncooked brown rice

Heat the oil in a large saucepan over a medium heat. Cook the onions and peppers until tender. Stir in the garlic when nearly done.

Add the passata, vegetable stock, black pepper and chilli powder. Reduce the heat to low and simmer, uncovered, for 20 minutes.

Add the rice, cover, and simmer for another 40 minutes until the rice is tender. Finally, stir in the peanut butter until well blended. Serve.

Cauliflower Cheese Soup

Easier and quicker to make than cauliflower cheese, this soup still has that lovely flavour. It's rich, creamy and filling but reasonably low in calories.

<u>Serves 6</u>   <u>Prep time 5m</u>   <u>Cook time 40m</u>

1 onion, finely chopped
1 cauliflower, cut into florets
1 small potato, chopped
700ml vegetable stock
400ml milk
100g mature cheddar, diced
1 knob of butter

Heat the butter in a large saucepan. Put in the onion and cook until it's soft - about 5 minutes. Add the cauliflower, potato, vegetable stock and milk. Bring to the boil, then reduce the heat and leave to simmer for about 30 minutes until the cauliflower is soft and the potato is turning to mush.

Whisk the mixture in a blender or food processor until you get a creamy, thick soup. Add more milk to thin a little if necessary.

When ready to serve, top with the cheese pieces, then stir through before eating.

Oriental Prawn Soup

A quick and spicy wok-based soup means one pan, zero fuss and supper's on the table in 10 minutes.

<u>Serves 4</u> <u>Prep time 0m</u> <u>Cook time 10m</u>

1 tbsp olive oil
300g bag of stir-fry vegetables
140g shiitake mushroom, sliced
2 tbsp Thai green curry paste
400g can coconut milk
200ml vegetable or fish stock
300g straight-to-wok medium noodles
200g raw prawns
2 sprigs of parsley, chopped

Heat the olive oil in the wok, then add and stir-fry the vegetables and the mushrooms for 2-3 minutes. Remove from the wok and put to one side.

Put the curry paste into the wok and fry for 1 min.

Pour in the coconut milk and stock. Bring to the boil, drop in the noodles and prawns, then reduce the heat and simmer for 4 minutes until the prawns are cooked through. Stir in the vegetables, mushrooms and the chopped parsley.

The soup is now ready to serve.

Snacks

Cheesy Crisps 102
Pork & Pear Sausage Rolls 103
Quinoa Muffins 104
Feta Fritters 105
Lemon Houmous 106
Squash Chunks 107
Chicken Satay Pieces.. 108
Salmon Mayonnaise Wraps 109
Stuffed Mushrooms 110

Cheesy Crisps

A quick, easy and much healthier take on shop-bought crisps. They taste a lot better too!

Makes 8 **Prep time 5m** **Cook time 10m**

100g parmesan cheese, grated
100g cheddar cheese, grated
100g ground almonds
2 tbsp olive oil

Preheat the oven to 150°C. Then line a baking tray with greaseproof paper.

Place both cheeses, the almonds and the olive oil in a bowl and mix together thoroughly. When done, spoon eight dollops of the mixture into the baking tray.

Cook in the oven for about 10 minutes until they are starting to go brown at the edges. Then remove them and allow to cool.

Your cheesy crisps are now ready to eat.

Pork & Pear Sausage Rolls

An unusual variation of the ever popular sausage roll. Here, we've used a pear but any hard fruit, such as an apple, will be just as good.

<u>Makes 6</u>   <u>Prep time 15m</u>   <u>Cook time 20m</u>

1 onion, diced
1 large pear, cored and finely chopped
3 sprigs of rosemary, chopped
500g pork, minced
½ tsp mustard seeds
500g puff pastry
1 egg

Put the pork, onion, pear, rosemary and mustard seeds in a blender and blitz to a fine paste. Put to one side.

Roll out the pastry to a 1/2cm thick rectangle. Cut it in half and put a strip of the pork paste down the centre of each half.

Beat the egg in a small bowl and then brush the edges of the pastry with the egg. Roll up both strips of pastry and brush on the rest of the beaten egg. Finally, cut each strip into three rolls.

Score the top of each roll and then place them in an oven set to 200°C. Bake for about 20 minutes.

Quinoa Muffins

High in protein, these savoury muffins with quinoa and feta cheese can be eaten either hot or cold.

Makes 8 **Prep time 10m** **Cook time 25m**

1 tbsp olive oil
1 small onion, chopped
1 clove of garlic, crushed
50g kale, finely chopped
3 eggs
250g quinoa, cooked
100g almonds, ground
50g feta cheese

Preheat the oven to 180°C.

Line a muffin tray with paper muffin cases and grease them with olive oil.

Beat the eggs in a bowl. Then add the onion, garlic, kale, quinoa and ground almonds. Crumble in the feta cheese, mix thoroughly and season to taste.

Spoon the mixture evenly into the muffin cases and bake for 20-25 minutes or until golden brown.

Feta Fritters

These courgette and feta fritters can be eaten as a snack, a starter or even a light meal.

<u>Serves 4</u>	<u>Prep time 5m</u>	<u>Cook time 5m</u>

3 courgettes, grated
1 lemon, grated zest of
1 red chilli, de-seeded and finely chopped
1 bunch of fresh mint, finely sliced
1 egg
25g plain flour
20g parmesan cheese
1 tsp oregano
100g feta cheese
1 tbsp olive oil

Beat the egg in a bowl and then add the courgette, flour, lemon zest, parmesan cheese, chilli, mint and oregano. Mix thoroughly and then crumble in the feta cheese and mix again.

Heat the olive oil in a frying pan and fry tablespoons of the mixture for a couple of minutes on each side until golden. Remove from the pan and serve.

Lemon Houmous

Houmous is so easy to make and beats shop-bought versions every time.

Serves 6 **Prep time 15m** **Cook time 0m**

2 400g cans chickpeas, drained
2 garlic cloves, finely chopped
3 tbsp yogurt
3 tbsp Tahini paste
3 tbsp olive oil
2 lemons, zest and juice of
20g coriander
Salt and pepper

Put everything but the coriander into a blender, then whisk to a smooth consistency.

Remove from the blender and place in a bowl. Season the houmous with the salt and pepper and then add the coriander.

Spoon it into a serving bowl, drizzle with the olive oil and serve.

Squash Chunks

Chunky wedges of squash covered in a crispy, spicy coating of nuts and seeds. Extremely nutritious.

<u>Serves 4</u>   <u>Prep time 10m</u>   <u>Cook time 45m</u>

50g hazelnuts
1 tbsp coriander seeds
2 tbsp sesame seeds
1 tbsp ground cumin
1 large butternut squash
1 tbsp olive oil

Preheat the oven to 200°C.

Toast the hazelnuts in a frying pan over a medium heat until golden. Add the coriander and sesame seeds, and toast for 1 minute more. Set aside. When cool, place in a blender together with the ground cumin and whisk until thoroughly mixed.

Peel the butternut squash, remove the seeds and slice into chunks. Toss the chunks with the olive oil, then cover them with the nut and seed coating.

Line a baking tray with greaseproof paper and add the coated chunks in a single layer. Cook for 30-40 minutes, turning halfway through, until tender.

Chicken Satay Pieces

Keep these nutty chicken satay strips in the fridge for a healthy option when you're feeling a bit peckish.

<u>Serves 2</u>   <u>Prep time 15m</u>   <u>Cook time 10m</u>

2 tbsp chunky peanut butter
1 garlic clove, finely grated
1 tsp Madras curry powder
1 tbsp soy sauce
2 tsp lime juice
2 chicken breast fillets cut into thick strips
15cm cucumber, cut into fingers
Sweet chilli sauce

Preheat the oven to 200°C.

Place the peanut butter, garlic, curry powder, soy sauce and lime juice in a bowl and mix well. If necessary, add a splash of boiling water to achieve the thickish consistency necessary for coating.

Add the chicken strips to the bowl and mix thoroughly ensuring they are well coated. Then place the strips in a baking tin lined with greaseproof paper and cook in the oven for about 10 minutes.

Eat with the cucumber fingers and chilli sauce.

Salmon Mayonnaise Wraps

Packed with omega-3-rich salmon, these delicious wraps with avocado and mayonnaise are an extremely healthy low-carb, high-protein snack.

Serves 2   Prep time 10m   Cook time 8m

1 tsp olive oil
2 salmon fillets
1 avocado
½ tsp English mustard powder
1 tsp cider vinegar
1 tbsp capers
8 lettuce leaves
16 cherry tomatoes, halved

Brush the salmon fillets with some olive oil, put them into a pan and cook for 3-4 minutes on each side.

Scoop the avocado's meat into a bowl. Add the mustard powder and vinegar, then mash well so that the mixture has a smooth mayonnaise-like consistency. Stir in the capers. Spoon into two small dishes and put on serving plates with the lettuce leaves and tomatoes.

Slice the salmon and arrange on the plates. Spoon some of the 'mayonnaise' onto the lettuce leaves and top with salmon and cherry tomatoes. To eat, roll up the lettuce leaves into little wraps.

Stuffed Mushrooms

Mushrooms stuffed with blue cheese, bacon, onions and garlic make a delicious and very nutritious snack.

<u>Serves 4</u>　　　<u>Prep time 15m</u>　　　<u>Cook time 35m</u>

4 strips bacon
4 large mushrooms
1 tbsp butter
1 tsp olive oil
1 small onion, diced
100g cream cheese
100g blue cheese

Preheat the oven to 175°C.

Fry the bacon in the olive oil and put it to one side. Remove the stems from the mushrooms and chop them up. Put the caps to one side.

Put the butter in a pan with the mushroom stems and onion. Cook them for about 15 minutes, stirring frequently, until the onion stems caramelise. Then put the onion and mushroom mixture into a blender together with the bacon, cream cheese and blue cheese. Blend to a smooth consistency.

Stuff the mixture into the mushroom caps and put them in a baking tin lined with greaseproof paper. Bake in the oven for 15 minutes.

Desserts

Coconut Macaroons 112

Chocolate & Peanut Squares 113

Blueberry Ice Cream 114

Chocolate Fudge 115

Pumpkin Pie 116

Saffron Pannacotta 117

Berry Crumble.. 118

Lemon Squares 119

Coconut Macaroons

This recipe does include a natural sweetener, but it can be reduced or even eliminated if desired. Either way, the macaroons are a very light yet satisfying dessert.

<u>Serves 2</u>   <u>Prep time 10m</u>   <u>Cook time 45m</u>

4 egg whites
4 tbsp honey
2 tsp vanilla extract
250g desiccated coconut
1 tbsp coconut oil
1 pinch of salt
75g dark chocolate

Preheat the oven to 160°C.

Whisk the egg whites with the salt until stiff. Then add the honey, vanilla, desiccated coconut and coconut oil, and mix with the egg whites.

Using a tablespoon, put large dollops of the macaroon mixture into a baking tin lined with greaseproof paper. Then bake them for about 15 minutes until they are just starting to turn brown. Remove from the oven.

Finally, melt the dark chocolate and then drizzle it over the cooked macaroons.

Chocolate & Peanut Squares

Chocolate and peanut butter could have been made for each other! The nuts give added crunchiness.

<u>Serves 4</u>   <u>Prep time 15m</u>   <u>Cook time 0m</u>

100g dark chocolate (cocoa content of at least 70%)
4 tbsp coconut oil
4 tbsp peanut butter
½ teaspoon vanilla extract
1 tsp ground cinnamon
4 tbsp peanuts, finely chopped
1 pinch salt

Melt the chocolate and coconut oil in a pan. Then add the salt, peanut butter, vanilla and cinnamon, and mix thoroughly.

Pour the batter into a small baking tin lined with greaseproof paper.

Let it cool for a while and then top with the chopped peanuts. Refrigerate.

When the batter is set, cut it into small squares. Store the chocolate and peanut squares in the refrigerator.

Blueberry Ice Cream

This blueberry ice cream is rich, creamy and delicious. Plus, you don't need an ice cream maker to make it!

Serves 6 **Prep time 90m** **Cook time 0m**

150g heavy whipping cream
3 egg yolks
½ tsp vanilla
½ tsp ground cardamom
½ lemon, zest of
225g mascarpone cheese
150g blueberries

Put the cream in a bowl and whip it until soft peaks form. Put it to one side.

In a separate bowl, add the egg yolks, vanilla, lemon zest and cardamom, and beat until fluffy. Mix in the mascarpone cheese and then add the whipped cream.

Add the blueberries to the mixture and combine well. Then pour it into a lidded container and place it in the freezer.

Stir the ice cream thoroughly every fifteen minutes until it firms up. This will take about 90 minutes.

Chocolate Fudge

A creamy low-carb fudge that is great as a small, but delicious, dessert. Add extra flavours if you want to, or serve as it is.

<u>Serves 6</u>   <u>Prep time 10m</u>   <u>Cook time 35m</u>

100g dark chocolate (cocoa content of at least 70%)
200g heavy whipping cream
1 tsp vanilla extract
75g butter

Boil the cream and vanilla in a pan for one minute and then lower to a simmer. Leave it simmering for 30 minutes. Then add the butter and mix into a smooth batter.

Remove from the heat and add pieces of the chocolate. Stir until the chocolate has melted into the batter. Add additional flavouring at this stage if so desired.

Pour the batter into a medium size baking tin and let it cool in the refrigerator for a couple of hours. Then take it out and sprinkle cocoa powder on top. Cut the fudge into pieces and serve cold.

Pumpkin Pie

Sweet pumpkin, succulent coconut and a kiss of lemon, all enveloped in a creamy filling. What could be nicer!

<u>Serves 6</u>   <u>Prep time 10m</u>   <u>Cook time 45m</u>

1 tbsp butter
4 tbsp shredded coconut
450g pumpkin
100g heavy whipping cream
¼ tsp salt
2 tsp pumpkin pie spice
1 lemon, zest of
1 tsp baking powder
3 eggs

Dice the pumpkin into cubes and place in a pan. Add the whipping cream, butter and salt, and bring to the boil. Then reduce the heat and let it simmer for 20 minutes until the pumpkin is soft. At this point, add the rest of the ingredients, except for the eggs, and blend to a smooth purée using a blender/food processor.

Beat the eggs in a bowl and then add the pumpkin purée and mix well.

Preheat the oven to 200°C. Grease a baking dish with butter and line it with the coconut flakes. Then pour the batter into the baking dish and bake for 20 minutes.

Saffron Pannacotta

A bright yellow and extremely delicious dessert, this low-carb pannacotta is very easy to make.

<u>Serves 6</u>   <u>Prep time 10m</u>   <u>Cook time 15m</u>

½ tbsp unflavoured powdered gelatin water
300g heavy whipping cream
¼ tsp vanilla extract
1 pinch saffron
1 tbsp almonds, chopped
12 raspberries

Mix the gelatin with water (follow the instructions on the pack) and set aside.

In a pan, boil the cream, vanilla and saffron. Lower the heat and allow to simmer for 10 minutes.

Remove the pan from the heat and add the gelatin. Stir until completely dissolved.

Pour the pannacotta mixture into 6 glasses. Cover the top of the glasses with plastic wrap and put them in the refrigerator for at least 2 hours.

Toast the almonds in a dry, hot, frying pan for a few minutes and then put them on top of the glasses of pannacotta together with the raspberries. Serve.

Berry Crumble

This scrumptious dessert is low in carbs, sugar-free, gluten-free and can be made without added sweeteners.

<u>Serves 4</u>   <u>Prep time 5m</u>   <u>Cook time 15m</u>

1 tsp coconut oil
300g mixed berries
150g almonds
75g pecans
2 tbsp butter
1 tsp cinnamon
1 tsp vanilla extract
1/4 tsp salt
5-10 drops liquid stevia sweetener (optional)

To make the berry base, heat the coconut oil in a pan then add the berries and cook them for 3-5 minutes.

To make the crumble, put the almonds and pecans in a food processor. Add the butter, cinnamon, vanilla, salt and stevia (if using). Pulse for a few seconds until the mixture is chopped to a fine consistency.

Sprinkle the nut mixture on top of the berries and cook for 10 minutes in an oven preheated to 200°C. Remove from the oven and serve.

Lemon Squares

These lemon squares don't just taste delicious, they are also very healthy.

<u>Serves 4</u>   <u>Prep time 5m</u>   <u>Cook time 15m</u>

150g almond flour, ground
1/4 tsp salt
1 tbsp coconut oil, melted
2 tbsp butter, melted
1 tbsp pure vanilla extract
1 tbsp honey
4 eggs
2 tbsp lemon juice

Preheat the oven to 175°C. Then line a medium size baking tin with greaseproof paper.

To make the crust, put the almond flour, salt, coconut oil, butter and vanilla extract in a bowl and mix it all thoroughly into a dough.

Press the dough evenly into the bottom of the baking tin. Bake it for about 15 minutes until lightly brown.

While the crust is baking, prepare the topping. In a blender or food processor (or by hand with a whisk), mix the almond flour, honey, eggs and lemon juice to a smooth consistency.

Cont'd

Remove the crust from the oven and pour the topping evenly all over it. Then return it to the oven and bake for another 15 minutes until the topping is brown at edges.

Remove from the oven and let it cool. Then refrigerate for 2 hours to let it set. Cut into squares and serve.

Nutritional Value of Fresh Fruit

	Calories	Fiber	Fat	Protein	Carbs
Apple - 1 medium	95	4.5g	0.5g	0.5g	25g
Apricot - 1 medium	14	0.5g	0g	0.5g	3g
Banana - 1 medium	105	3g	0.5g	1.5g	27g
Blackberry - 1 cup	62	7.5g	0.5g	2g	14g
Blueberry - 1 cup	83	3.5g	0.5g	1g	21g
Cherry - 1 cup	74	2.5g	0g	1g	19g
Coconut meat - 1 cup	283	7g	27g	2.5g	12g
Cranberry - 1 cup	60	4g	0g	0g	10g
Dates - 1 cup	495	15g	0g	4g	133g
Elderberry - 1 cup	106	10g	0.5g	1g	27g
Figs - 1 cup	492	20g	2g	6g	127g
Grapes - 1 cup	110	1g	0g	1g	27g
Grapefruit - 1 medium	82	3g	0g	1.5g	20g
Guava - 1 medium	61	5g	1g	2.5g	13g
Kiwi - 1 medium	42	2g	0.5g	1g	10g
Lemon - 1 medium	17	1.5g	0g	0.5g	5.5g
Lime - 1 medium	20	2g	0g	0.5g	7g
Mango - 1 medium	145	3.5g	0.5g	1g	35g
Mulberry - 1 cup	60	2.5g	0.5g	2g	14g
Orange - 1 medium	62	3g	0g	1g	15g
Papaya - 1 cup	60	2.5g	0.5g	0.5g	16g
Passion Fruit - 1 med	5	0.5g	0.5g	0.5g	1g
Peach - 1 medium	38	1.5g	0g	1g	9g
Pear - 1 medium	96	5g	0g	0.5g	25g
Plum - 1 medium	20	0.5g	0g	0.5g	5g
Pineapple - 1 cup	82	2.5g	0g	1g	21g
Pomegranate - 1 med	100	1g	0.5g	1g	26g
Raspberry - 1 cup	64	8g	1g	1.5g	15g
Rhubarb - 1 cup	26	2g	0g	1g	5.5g
Strawberry - 1 cup	49	3g	0.5g	1g	12g
Watermelon - 1 cup	45	0.5g	0g	1g	11g

Nutritional Value of Dried Fruit

	Calories	Fiber	Fat	Protein	Carbs
Apple - 1 cup	240	6g	0g	1g	50g
Apricots - 1 cup	310	9.5g	0.5g	4.5g	82g
Cranberries - 1 cup	520	8g	0g	0g	136g
Dates - 1 cup	493	15g	0g	4g	133g
Figs - 1 cup	490	20g	2g	6g	127g
Goji Berries - 1 cup	300	2g	3g	18g	60g
Prunes - 1 cup	408	12g	0.5g	3.5g	109g
Raisins - 1 cup	436	5g	1g	4g	115g
Sultanas - 1 cup	656	4.5g	0g	4.5g	154g

Nutritional Value of Fruit Juices

	Calories	Fiber	Fat	Protein	Carbs
Apple - 1 cup	117	0g	0.5g	0g	29g
Beetroot - 1 cup	96	0g	0g	3g	21g
Carrot - 1 cup	80	0g	0g	2g	17g
Cranberry - 1 cup	110	0g	0g	0g	28g
Grapefruit - 1 cup	96	0g	0g	1g	23g
Lemon - 1 tablespoon	3	0g	0g	0g	1g
Lime - 1 tablespoon	5	0g	0g	0g	1.5g
Orange - 1 cup	112	0.5g	0.5g	1.5g	26g
Pineapple - 1 cup	120	0g	0g	0g	31g
Pomegranate - 1 cup	100	0g	0g	0g	20g
Prune - 1cup	180	2.5g	0g	1.5g	45g
Tomato - 1 cup	41	1g	0g	2g	10g
Coconut water - 1 cup	46	2.5g	0.5g	1.5g	9g

Nutritional Value of Vegetables

	Calories	Fiber	Fat	Protein	Carbs
Artichoke - 1 medium	60	7g	0g	4g	13g
Asparagus - 1 cup	27	3g	0g	3g	5g
Avocado - 1 medium	289	12g	26.5g	3.5g	15g
Beetroot - 1 medium	35	2.5g	0g	1.5g	8g
Broccoli - 1 cup	31	2.5g	0.5g	2.5g	6g
Brussels Sprouts - 1 cup	38	3.5g	0.5g	3g	8g
Cabbage - 1 cup	22	2g	0g	1g	5g
Carrots - 1 medium	25	1.5g	0g	0.5g	6g
Cauliflower - 1 cup	25	2.5g	0g	2g	5.5g
Celery - 1 stalk	6	0.5g	0g	0.5g	1g
Courgette - 1 medium	40	2g	1g	3.5g	5g
Cucumber - 1 medium	24	1.5g	0.5g	1g	4.5g
Eggplant - 1 medium	21	3g	0.5g	1g	5g
Fennel - 1 medium	73	7g	0.5g	3g	17g
Ginger - 1 teaspoon	1.5	1g	0g	0g	1g
Green Beans - 1 cup	34	3.5g	0g	2g	8g
Kale - 1 cup	33	1g	1g	0.5g	7g
Lettuce - 1 cup	10	0g	0g	1g	2g
Mushrooms - 1 cup	15	1g	0g	2g	2g
Onion - 1 medium	47	2.5g	0g	1.5g	10g
Parsnip - 1 cup	100	6g	0.5g	1.5g	24g
Pepper - 1 medium	30	2g	0g	1g	8g
Potato - 1 medium	164	4.5g	0g	4g	37g
Pumpkin - 1 medium	30g	0.5g	0g	1g	7.5g
Radish - 1 cup	13	1g	0g	1g	4g
Spinach - 1 cup	7	1g	0g	1g	1g
Squash - 1 cup	18	1g	0g	1.5g	4g
Sweet Potato - 1 med	112	4g	0g	3g	26g
Tomato - 1 medium	22	1.5g	0g	1g	5g
Turnip - 1 medium	34	2g	0g	1g	8g
Watercress - 1 cup	7	0.5g	0g	1g	0g
Zucchini - 1 medium	32	2g	0.5g	2.5g	6.5g

Nutritional Value of Nuts

	Calories	Fiber	Fat	Protein	Carbs
Almonds - 1 cup	823	17.5g	71g	30g	31g
Brazil - 1 cup	920	10g	93g	20g	17g
Cashews - 1 cup	960	4g	76g	28g	44g
Chestnuts - 1 cup	210	2g	2g	4g	44g
Coconut - 1 cup	490	14g	50g	7g	8g
Hazelnuts - 1 cup	720	8g	72g	16g	16g
Macadamia - 1 cup	961	11g	101g	10.5g	18.5g
Peanuts - 1 cup	825	12g	71g	38g	24g
Pecans - 1 cup	760	4g	80g	12g	16g
Pistachios - 1 cup	740	12g	52g	24g	36g
Walnuts - 1 cup	800	8g	80g	20g	16g

Nutritional Value of Seeds

	Calories	Fiber	Fat	Protein	Carbs
Chia - 1 tablespoon	67	5.5g	4.5g	3g	0.5g
Flax - 1 tablespoon	37	2g	2g	1.5g	2g
Hemp - 1 tablespoon	57	0.5g	4.5g	3.5g	0.5g
Linseeds - 1 tablespoon	49	2.5g	4g	1.5g	2.5g
Poppy - 1 tablespoon	47	1g	4g	1.5g	2g
Pumpkin - 1 tablespoon	56	0.5g	5g	3g	1g
Sesame - 1 tablespoon	52	1g	4.5g	1.5g	2g
Sunflower - 1 tablespoon	47	1g	4g	1.5g	2g

Nutritional Value of Pulses

	Calories	Fiber	Fat	Protein	Carbs
Blackeyed peas - 1 cup	200	8g	4g	12g	34g
Black beans - 1 cup	240	12g	1g	14g	46g
Broad beans - 1 cup	160	8g	0.5g	10g	28g
Butter beans - 1 cup	200	10g	0g	10g	38g
Chickpeas - 1 cup	210	7g	3g	11g	34g
Green Peas - 1 cup	117	7.5g	0.5g	8g	21g
Lentils - 1 cup	320	44g	0g	40g	80g
Mung beans - 1 cup	600	33g	1.5g	49g	110g
Pinto beans - 1 cup	670	30g	2.5g	41g	120g
Kidney beans - 1 cup	216	15.5g	0g	14g	43g
Soya beans - 1 cup	290	12g	14.5g	28g	10g
Split Peas - 1 cup	440	48g	0g	40g	112g

Nutritional Value of Misc

	Calories	Fiber	Fat	Protein	Carbs
Almond milk - 1 cup	60	0.5g	2.5g	0.5g	8g
Almond butter - 1 tbsp	102	0.5g	9g	3.5g	3g
Honey - 1 tbsp	70	0.5g	0g	0g	17g
Soya milk - 1 cup	132	1.5g	4.5g	8g	15.5g
Low-fat yoghurt - 1 cup	125	0g	2.5g	7g	19g
Low-fat milk - 1 cup	110	0g	2.5g	9g	13g
Protein powder - 1 tbsp	110	0g	1.5g	23g	1g
Peanut butter - 1 tbsp	94	1g	8g	4g	3g
Cinnamon - 1 teaspoon	6	1g	0g	0g	4g
Turmeric - 1 tbsp	24	1.5g	0.5g	1g	120g
Oats - 1 cup	166	4g	3.5g	6g	28g
Cod liver oil - 1 tbsp	135	0g	15g	0g	0g
Olive oil - 1 tbsp	120	0g	14g	0g	0g

Conversion Charts

Converting Liquid

US Cups	Metric	Imperial
1 cup	250 ml	8 fl oz
3/4 cup	180 ml	6 fl oz
2/3 cup	150 ml	5 fl oz
1/2 cup	120 ml	4 fl oz
1/3 cup	75 ml	2 1/2 fl oz
1/4 cup	60 ml	2 fl oz
1/8 cup	30 ml	1 fl oz
1 tablespoon	15 ml	1/2 fl oz
1 teaspoon	5 ml	1/6 fl oz

Converting Weight

US Cups	Metric	Imperial
1 cup	150 g	5 oz
3/4 cup	110 g	3 2/3 oz
2/3 cup	100 g	3 1/2 oz
1/2 cup	75 g	2 1/2 oz
1/3 cup	50 g	1 3/4 oz
1/4 cup	40 g	1 1/2 oz
1/8 cup	20 g	3/4 oz
1 tablespoon	10 g	1/3 oz
1 teaspoon	3 g	1/10 oz

Index

A

Almonds 23, 59, 70, 102, 104, 117
  Flour 59, 65
Apple 15, 19, 26, 57
Apricots 23
Aubergine 72
Avocado 32, 35, 87, 88, 109

B

Bacon 13, 22, 24, 90, 110
Baking powder 116
Bamboo shoots 30
Barbecue 57
Basil 12, 40, 56, 73
Bay leaves 68
BBQ 57
Beans
  Baked 24
  Black 85
  Broard 91
  Cannellini 14
  Chilli 92
  French 61
  Green 37, 56
  Kidney 92
Bean sprouts 81, 84
Beef 63, 68, 84
Beef stock 51
Beef stock cube 68
Black bean sauce 31

Black pudding 22
Blueberries 114
Braising steak 68
Breadcrumbs 13, 32
Broccoli 55
Bulgar mushroom 93
Burger 32
Burritos 29
Butter 13, 16, 20, 36, 65, 93, 99, 110, 115, 116, 118
Butternut squash 70

C

Cabbage 95
  Chinese 31
Cajun seasoning 50
Capers 109
Cardamom 114
Carrot 28, 34, 37, 43, 61, 74, 86, 95
Casserole 58
Cauliflower 21, 30, 37, 48, 67, 99
Celery 90, 91, 95
Cheese 12, 44, 99
  Blue 110
  cheddar 13, 99
  Cheddar 28, 54
  Cream 13, 28, 29, 59, 110
  Feta 78, 80, 82, 104
  Mascarpone 114
  Mozzarella 12, 59, 67, 72
  Parmesan 13, 72, 102, 105
Cheesy crisps 102
Chestnuts 70
Chicken 14, 29, 35, 46, 50, 53, 55, 65, 76, 81, 85, 96, 108
  Stock 50, 55, 93
  Stock cube 46

Chickpeas 33, 42, 83, 91, 106
Chilli 31, 39, 48, 58, 63, 81, 83
  Red 97, 105
  Scotch bonnet 46
  Flakes 84
  Paste 55
  Powder 29, 35, 42, 59, 76
  Sauce 40
Chinese five-spice powder 31, 63
Chocolate 113, 115
  Dark 112
Chorizo 50
Ciambotta 56
Cinnamon 15, 16, 92, 113
Coconut 112
  Desiccated 112
  Flour 65
  Milk 37, 97, 100
  Oil 113, 118
Coriander 31, 33, 35, 37, 43, 48, 91
Cornflour 34, 96
Courgette 18, 54, 61, 72, 86, 105
Couscous 79
Cranberries 70
Cream 73
  Sour 58, 93
  Whipping 114, 115, 117
Cucumber 43, 78, 81, 84, 88, 108
Cumin 21, 37, 42, 48, 53, 91, 92
Curry 37
  Paste 30

D

Dill 34, 93
Duck 31

E

Egg 14, 17, 18, 22, 25, 59, 70, 103, 105, 114
  Scrambled 20

F

Fajitas 76
Fennel 56, 74
Fish 74
  Cakes 43
  Farms 36
  Fillets 74
  Sauce 81
  Steamed 39
  Stock cube 74
Flour 63
  Almond 119
  Plain 93, 105
Food bag 57
Food processor 67, 95
Fritters 105
Fudge 115

G

Garam masala 53
Garlic 12, 14, 18, 25, 29, 33, 37, 44, 50, 53, 63, 80, 83, 92, 104
Gelatin water 117
Ginger 31, 36, 37, 43, 53, 63, 97
Goulash 68
Granola 16
Griddle pan 57

H

Haddock 21

Ham 13, 20
Hazelnuts 107
Hoisin sauce 55
Honey 16, 19, 23, 26, 112, 119
Horseradish sauce 32
Houmous 106

I

Ice cream 114

J

Jambalaya 50

K

Kale 104
Kedgeree 21
Konnyaku 47
Kugel 28

L

Lasagne 54
Leek 17, 52, 65, 74
Lemon 21, 36, 37, 42, 57, 76, 82, 93, 106, 119
  Balm 79
  Juice 33
  Zest 83, 91, 105, 114
Lentils 37, 90
Lettuce 81, 87, 88, 109
Lime 35, 39, 84, 97, 108
  Leaves 81
Linseed 26

M

Macaroons 112
Madras curry powder 108
Mayonnaise 86, 87, 109
Milk 15, 19, 20, 25, 93, 99
Mince meat 58, 59
Minestrone 95
Mint 79, 105
  Leaves 86
Muesli 19
Muffins 104
Mushroom 12, 13, 17, 20, 22, 24, 25, 33, 51, 73, 93, 110
  Shiitake 100
Mussel 74
Mustard 28, 88, 109
  Dijon 80, 86
  Seeds 103

N

Nachos 59
Noodles 100
  Egg 41
  Shirataki 40
Nutmeg 26, 48, 70
Nuts 70

O

Oats 23
  Rolled 19, 26
Oil
  Olive 17, 18, 29, 37, 56, 61, 68, 74, 82, 88, 91, 95, 104, 110
  Sesame 52, 96
  Sunflower 28
Okra 46
Old El Paso Fajita spice mix 85

Olives 51, 78, 80
Omelette 12
　Mushroom & garlic 25
Onion 12, 13, 14, 18, 24, 28, 37, 48, 61, 73, 78, 90, 93, 99
　Red 57, 86
　Spring 32, 55, 63, 84
Oregano 14, 51, 67, 72, 78, 105

P

Paella 61
Pak choi 31, 39
Pannacotta 117
Paprika 53, 61, 93
Parsley 32, 33, 61, 80, 83, 90, 100
Passata 14, 98
Pasta
　Penne 33
Pastry 103
Peanut 98, 113
　Butter 98, 108, 113
Pear 103
Pearl barley 73
Peas 30
　Frozen 61
　Sugar snap 31, 41
Pecans 118
Pepper 14, 18, 29, 35, 41, 50, 52, 68
　Black 13, 17, 82, 91
　Red 46, 72, 83, 98
　Sauce 76
　Yellow 46
Pilaf 44
Pineapple 30
Pine nuts 82
Pizza 67

133

Plaice 34
Pork 41, 103
  Steaks 57
Porridge 15
  Apple and linseed 26
  Oats 16
Potato 14, 24, 95, 99
Prawns 30, 48, 74, 100
Psyllium husk 65
Pumpkin 97, 116

Q

Quinoa 15, 44, 80, 104

R

Radish 86
Raisins 23
Raspberries 19, 117
Ratatouille 18
Red curry paste 43
Red wine 63
Rice 29, 30, 46
  Brown 98
  Shirataki 46, 50, 61
Ricotta 54
Risotto 73
Rocket 32
Rosemary 67, 103

S

Saffron 117
Salad 77
  Avocado and sunflower 87
  Chicken 81

  Couscous 79
  Fire 85
  Greek 78
  Greens 85
  Indian summer 86
  Lemon and Feta 82
  Quinoa 80
  Sausage 88
  Squid and pepper 83
  Vietnamese beef 84
Salmon 21, 32, 36, 43, 109
  Alaskan 36
  Atlantic 36
Salsa 85
Salt 37, 42, 65, 83, 93
Samphire 34
Satay 108
Sausage 22, 24, 51, 88
  Rolls 103
Seeds
  Sesame 16, 107
  Sunflower 15, 16, 44, 80, 87
Soup 90
  Cauliflower cheese 99
  Chicken 96
  Chickpea 91
  Chilli bean 92
  Lentil & bacon 90
  Minestrone 95
  Oriental prawn 100
  Oriental pumpkin 97
  Peanut 98
Soy sauce 36, 39, 43, 63, 76, 84, 93, 108
Spinach 14, 44, 48, 70, 82
Squash 107

Squid 83
Stevia 118
Stew 51, 74
Stock cube 73
Sugar 48, 97
  Brown 36
  Caster 43
  Muscovado 88
Sweetcorn 79, 84, 85, 96

T

Tabasco Sauce 13
Tahini 33
Tahini paste 106
Thai green curry paste 100
Thai red curry paste 97
Thyme 18
Tomato 12, 18, 20, 22, 24, 42, 46, 58, 78, 85
  Cherry 80, 88
  Chopped 61, 68
  Paste 58
  Plum 50, 91
  Purée 46, 68, 95
  Sauce 54
Tortilla 29, 35, 76
Tortilla chips 59
Turmeric 37, 48, 53, 61, 74

V

Vanilla 15, 112, 113, 118
Vegetable bouillon 33
Vegetable stock 37, 41, 61, 92, 97, 99
Venison 52
Vinegar 57

Balsamic 87
Cider 109
Red wine 87, 88
White wine 43, 86

W

Walnut 19
Worcestershire sauce 14, 76

Y

Yogurt 17, 19, 21, 106
  Greek 34, 53

Printed in Poland
by Amazon Fulfillment
Poland Sp. z o.o., Wrocław